11/30/2009
For Gabriele McLaughlin
Keep strong, fit + flexible

Ken Hanoey MD

Bloodless Spine Surgery

Pictures and Explanations

First Edition
Published by Dee Dee LLC.
ISBN 978-0-9745374-0-5
®2008 by Dee Dee LLC™

Kenneth K. Hansraj, M.D.
Orthopedic Surgery of The Spine
Work: 845-471-9200
Fax: 845-471-1551
Web: www.specialspine.com

This book is dedicated
to my mom,
Anjanie Devi Hansraj

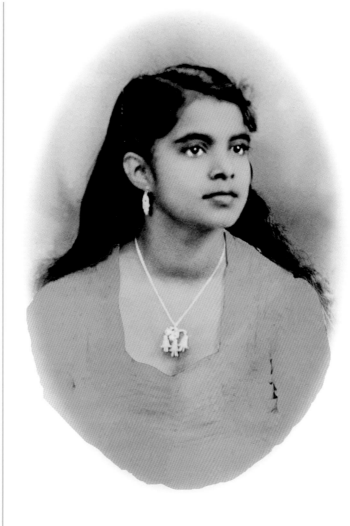

Contents

Acknowledgments

This book was produced with the encouragement of many. I wish to thank you all for your kindness.

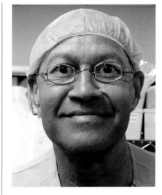

Basil S. Abeyasekera, M.D.

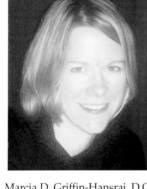

Marcia D. Griffin-Hansraj, D.O.

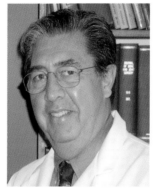

Gregory J. Chiaramonte, M.D.

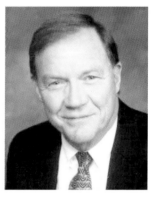

Robert Savage

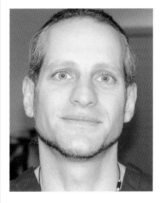

Baron Heisey, P.A.

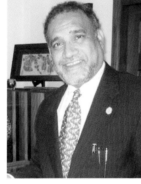

Harry Walia

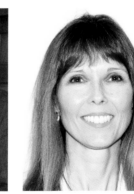

Gina Mandel, R.N.

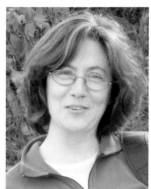

Marcy Decker

Special Thanks

Bloodless spine surgery is achievable only with a team effort. I am grateful to the team of anesthesiologists.

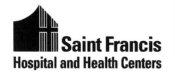
Saint Francis
Hospital and Health Centers

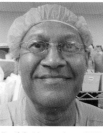
Basil S. Abeyasekera, M.D.

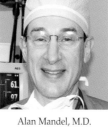
Alan Mandel, M.D.

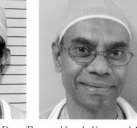
B.R. Mylar Rao, M.D.

Thummakkundu Venugopal, M.D.

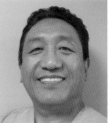
Lobsang T. Lhungay, M.D.

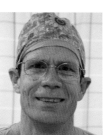
Paul Cooke, M.D.

Mohammed Siddidqui, M.D.

William N. Smookler, M.D.

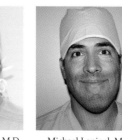
Michael Lapinel, M.D.

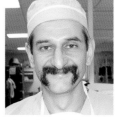
Victor Overtchenko, M.D.

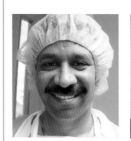
Nagendra Uphadyayula, M.D.

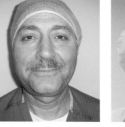
Leon A. Basil, M.D.

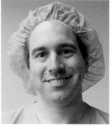
Robert E. Tomkins, D.O.

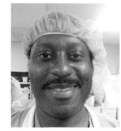
Harold E. Gardner, CRNA

Special Thanks

Our fine operating room personnel contributes significantly to successful surgeries.

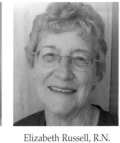
Patty Sullivan, R.N.

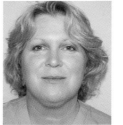
Elizabeth Russell, R.N.

Kellen Roberto, R.N.

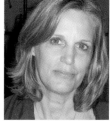
Theresa Bostock, R.N.

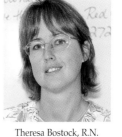
Barbara Covello, R.N.

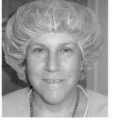
Kathleen Neumann, R.N.

Andrew Bounds, R.N.

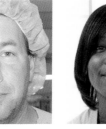
James Balint, R.N.

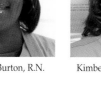
Maliuqka Burton, R.N.

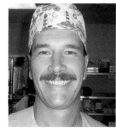
Kimberly Mihans, R.N.

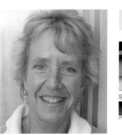
Caryn Solomon, R.N.

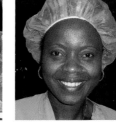
Deborah Kirstein, R.N.

Conceptor Orende, R.N.

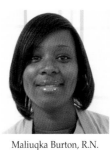
Gabrielle Berry, CRNFA

Kevin Dahowski, PCT

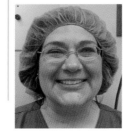
Geri Mortensen, ST

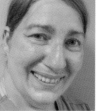
Cathy Meisner, CTS

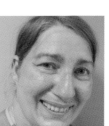
Carol Surico, ST

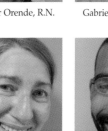
Eric Peterson, ST

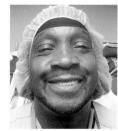
Rob Brewer, ST

Introduction

When a pitcher is training his shoulder, one would assume that the focus of the rehabilitation is the shoulder. However, time must also be spent on the abdominal muscles, back muscles, and lower extremity muscles, with special emphasis on the buttock muscles. Otherwise, there will be no foundation for performance.

Similarly, in preparing a patient for safe bloodless spine surgery, a comprehensive evaluation is recommended. This ensures no surprises in the operating room.

With the development of advanced decompression and instrumentation techniques with bone graft options, spine surgery is much more established and effective.

Safety remains the predominant concern. Blood transfusions have recognized risk factors. Bloodless is the goal, the destination, and quite possibly the dream. Realistically, however, blood will be lost in all surgeries. Nevertheless, surgeons will persist in rallying to lose the least amount of blood at every possible step. In this book, factors that govern blood loss and blood transfusion are discussed.

This book presents the comprehensive preparation of a patient for bloodless spine surgery, techniques for diminishing blood loss in the operating room, and postoperative considerations. It includes case reports of patients who have undergone surgery using the blood management methods outlined.

Considerations and choices for Jehovah's Witnesses are discussed. Witnesses will not accept whole blood, primary components (red cells, white cells, platelets and plasma) or fractions. Fractions are elements extracted from the primary components of blood and therefore may note be acceptable to a Jehovah's Witness.

Digital images and illustrations are incorporated throughout the book to show important concepts, and a dictionary is provided to thoroughly explain the important factors in bloodless surgery.

An effort was made to ensure that the information is clear to readers who come from a nonmedical background.

Common Spinal Conditions

Herniated Nucleus Pulposus

The normal disc is a combination of strong connective tissues that hold one vertebra to the next. This disc serves as a cushion. This human shock absorber called the disc consists of a tough outer layer called the annulus fibrosus and a gel-like center called the nucleus pulposus. A herniated disc exists when the nucleus pulposus exits through the annulus fibrosus.

Classically, the patient complains of back pain and a sharp, lancing pain progressing distally from groin/buttock/hip into the leg or arm in a specific zone. Radiculopathy refers to the irritation of a nerve root, causing symptoms (pain, numbness, weakness, and reflex changes) in the zone of the nerve root.

Numbness, tingling or weakness of the leg is called sciatica. Sciatica affects about 1–2% of all people, usually between the ages of 30 and 50. Similar symptoms may be experienced in the arms or around the trunk.

Loss of bowel or bladder control is an emergency. Seek immediate medical attention!

Traditional treatments include short term bed rest, traction, physical therapy, massages, modalities (ice, heat, tens/sequential stimulation, ultrasound), acupuncture, osteopathy, chiropractic care, pain management (epidural versus super selective nerve root blocks), activity avoidance, activity and job modifications. Heat (in the form of long hot showers, sauna, and hot water bottles) may be helpful. Application of cold packs and gels may also relieve pain. Medications in the classes of aspirin, nonsteroidal anti-inflammatories, muscle relaxants, oral steroids, antidepressants and narcotics may be recommended. External stabilization in the form of a brace may be helpful.

When the patient is less symptomatic, specific stabilization such as cervical or lumbar stabilization may assist the patient to resume function and endurance. Pilates may be used to strengthen core abdominal muscles, while Medx treatment may strengthen trunk extensors.

Cervical spine (neck) surgical treatments include anterior cervical discectomy and fusion (ACDF) and posterior foraminotomy with discectomy.

Thoracic spine (midback) surgical treatments include posterior decompression by costotransversectomy and anterior decompression by thoracotomy. Fusion stabilization may also be necessary.

Lumbar spine (lower back) surgical treatments include standard discectomy, microdiscetomy, endoscopic discectomy, and percutaneous discectomy. At times surgical stabilization in the form of spinal fusion may be recommended.

Prevention: While the process of wear, tear and breakdown of discs is natural and unavoidable, certain factors accelerate the process. Repetitive bending, lifting, twisting, reaching, vibration exposure, poor posture, poor body mechanics, weak abdominal and lumbar extensor muscles, smoking and obesity may increase the rate of disc breakdown.

Herniated Disc

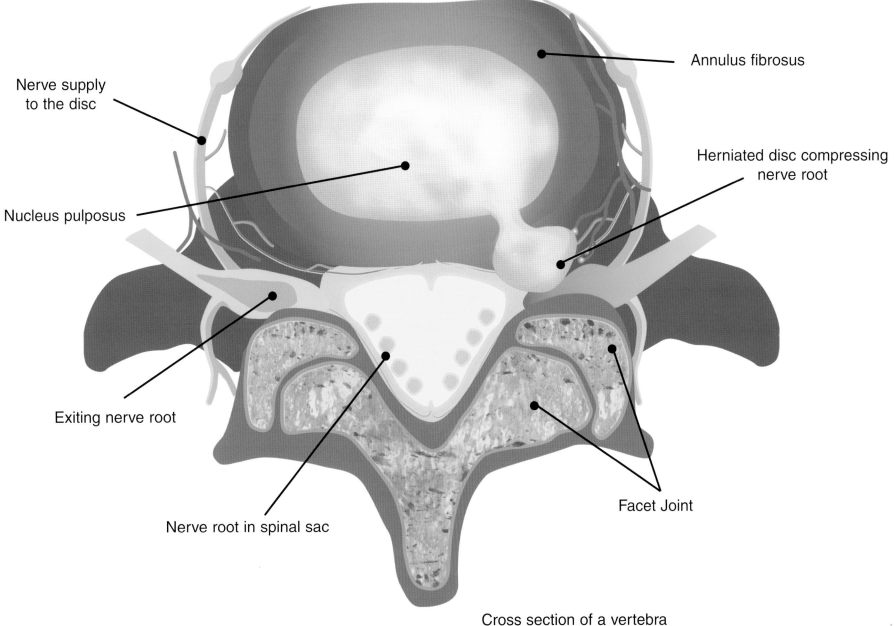

Annulus fibrosus

Nerve supply to the disc

Herniated disc compressing nerve root

Nucleus pulposus

Exiting nerve root

Facet Joint

Nerve root in spinal sac

Cross section of a vertebra

Degenerative Disc Disease

Degenerative disc disease represent the wear and tear to the human shock absorber called the disc. This process happens naturally with aging. However, it may be accelerated with trauma such as motor vehicle accidents, or work and repetitive activities. It is recognized that the degenerative disc causes pain by spilling inflammatory chemicals that are caustic to nerve roots and neural elements.

Classically, the patient complains of back pain worsened with sitting and standing. This pain is commonly reported to be a deep boring pain progressing distally from the groin/ buttock/hip into the leg or arm in a nonspecific zone. Numbness, tingling or weakness of the leg is called sciatica. Sciatica affects about 1–2% of all people, usually between the ages of 30 and 50. Similar symptoms may be experienced in the arms or around the trunk. Radiculopathy refers to the irritation of a nerve root, causing symptoms (pain, numbness, weakness, and reflex changes) in the zone of the nerve root.

Loss of bowel or bladder control is an emergency. Seek immediate medical attention!

Traditional treatments include short term bed rest, traction, physical therapy, massages, modalities (ice, heat, tens/sequential stimulation, ultrasound), acupuncture, osteopathy, chiropractic care, pain management (epidural versus super selective nerve root blocks, facet blocks or radiofrequency ablation), activity avoidance, activity and job modifications. Heat (in the form of long hot showers, sauna, and hot water bottles) may be helpful. Application of cold packs and gels may also relieve pain. Medications in the classes of aspirin, non-steroidal anti-inflammatories, muscle relaxants, oral steroids, anti-depressants and narcotics may be recommended. External stabilization in the form of a brace may be helpful.

When the patient is less symptomatic, specific stabilization such as cervical or lumbar stabilization may assist the patient to resume function and endurance. Pilates may be used to strengthen core abdominal muscles, while Medx treatment may strengthen trunk extensors.

Minimally invasive surgical treatments include thermodiskoplasty, IDET, and nucleoplasty.

Surgical treatments include posterior spinal fusion with instrumentation, posterior lumbar interbody fusion (PLIF), transforminal lumbar interbody fusion (TLIF), anterior spinal fusion, anterior spinal fusion and posterior spinal fusion and disk replacement.

Prevention: While the process of wear, tear and breakdown of discs is natural and unavoidable, certain factors accelerate the process. Repetitive bending, lifting, twisting, reaching, vibration exposure, poor posture, poor body mechanics, weak abdominal and lumbar extensor muscles, smoking and obesity may increase the rate of disc breakdown.

Normal Disc

Degenerative Disc

The wear and tear to the human shock absorber are represented by these rips and tears in the disc. Chemicals known as inflammatory factors are noted to leak from these rips and tears.

Spinal Stenosis

Spinal stenosis occurs when arthritic build-up blocks the spinal channels. This causes a narrowing of the spinal canal and/or nerve canal. The two main channels are the central canal, which carries the spinal cord, and the nerve canal (neuroforamen). With activity, time, wear and tear, arthritic spurs build up on the facet joints in the posterior part of the spine. These arthritic spurs then encroach on the nerve channel and pinch the nerve roots. This may occur in the neck (cervical), mid-back (thoracic) and lower back (lumbar).

Classically, with cervical stenosis patients may present with nerve root symptoms when the nerve roots are compressed. When the spinal cord is compressed, the patient may have lower greater than upper extremity weakness, a broad-based shuffling gait, incoordination of one or both limbs, difficulty knowing where a limb is in space, numbness in the lower extremities, radiating lightning-like sensations down the back with neck flexion and rarely bowel and bladder changes.

Classically, with lumbar spinal stenosis, patients complain of pain in the back, sciatic-type pain in the legs, pain on standing with relief by lying/sitting down, cramping and pain in calves with walking short distances, greater ease walking uphill than walking downhill, the ability to ride a bike with ease, often over long distances. Spinal or nerve claudication refers to pain in the legs, the calves, or the buttocks that is associated with activity. The pain is often relieved by sitting and resting, and it starts up again with activity.

The shopping cart sign is when patients report that they are able to walk long distances holding on to a shopping cart. Typically they are stooped over, opening the lumbar spinal channels a bit.

In the cervical spine the bottom two levels (C5-6 and C6-7) are most commonly involved. In the lumbar spine spinal stenosis is most common in the L3-4, L4-5. It is diagnosed and confirmed by an MRI or CAT scan/myelogram.

Traditional treatments include short bed rest, traction, physical therapy, massages, modalities (ice, heat, tens/sequential stimulation, ultrasound), acupuncture, osteopathy, chiropractic care, pain management (epidural versus super selective nerve root blocks), activity avoidance, activity and job modifications. Medications in the classes of aspirin, nonsteroidal anti-inflammatories, muscle relaxants, oral steroids, anti-depressants and narcotics may be recommended.

In the cervical spine decompressive procedures may be recommended from the front or back of the spine, depending on where the narrowing is. Stabilization/fusion may be recommended at the same time.

Pilates may be used to strengthen core abdominal muscles, while Medx treatment may strengthen trunk extensors.

Lumbar surgical treatments include decompression, as well as decompression fusion and instrumentation. At times anterior surgical stabilization may be recommended.

Prevention: While the process of wear, tear and breakdown of discs is natural and unavoidable, certain factors accelerate the process. Repetitive bending, lifting, twisting, reaching, vibration exposure, poor posture, poor body mechanics, weak abdominal and lumbar extensor muscles, smoking and obesity may increase the rate of disc breakdown and therefore arthritis formation.

Central Spinal Stenosis

Lateral Spinal Stenosis

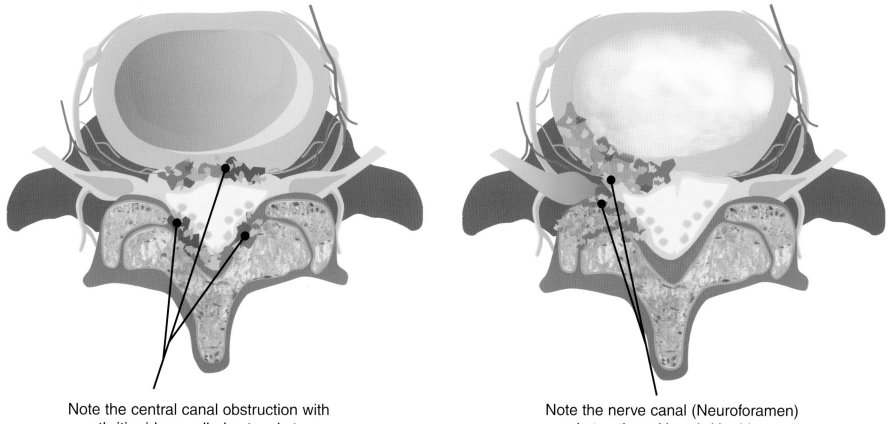

Note the central canal obstruction with arthritic ridges called osteophytes

Note the nerve canal (Neuroforamen) obstruction with arthritic ridges

Spondylolisthesis is a condition in which one vertebral body is slipped over the other (spondylos = vertebra, olisthesis = to slip). Leon Wiltse and colleagues devised a classification system:

Type	Classification	Caused by:
1	Dysplastic	Genetics – born with it
2	Isthmic	Lesion located in the pars interarticularis
3	Degenerative	Degenerative arthritis and instability of the facet joints with an intact neural arch
4	Traumatic	Trauma, e.g., MVA, fall
5	Pathologic	Tumor
6	Postsurgical	Removing bone, as in decompression

Spondylolisthesis may be further classified by:

Grade	% Slip
1	1–24%
2	25–49%
3	50–74%
4	75–99%
5	100%*

*Called spondyloptosis

Classically, patients complain of back pain and a dull pain progressing distally from the buttock especially into the posterior thigh. Some patients report hamstring tightness, spasm and pain. Others have no symptoms. In advanced cases the patient has a swayback with a protruding abdomen, exhibits a shortened torso, and presents with a waddling gait.

Traditional treatments include short bed rest, traction, physical therapy, massages, modalities (ice, heat, tens/sequential stimulation, ultrasound), acupuncture, osteopathy, chiropractic care, pain management (epidural versus super selective nerve root blocks), activity avoidance, activity and job modifications. Medications in the classes of aspirin, non-steroidal anti-inflammatories, muscle relaxants, oral steroids, anti-depressants and narcotics may be recommended.

External stabilization in the form of a brace may be helpful.

When the patient is less symptomatic, lumbar stabilization may assist the patient to resume function and endurance. Pilates may be used to strengthen core abdominal muscles, while Medx treatment may strengthen trunk extensors.

Surgical treatments include decompression, as well as decompression fusion and instrumentation. At times anterior surgical stabilization may be recommended.

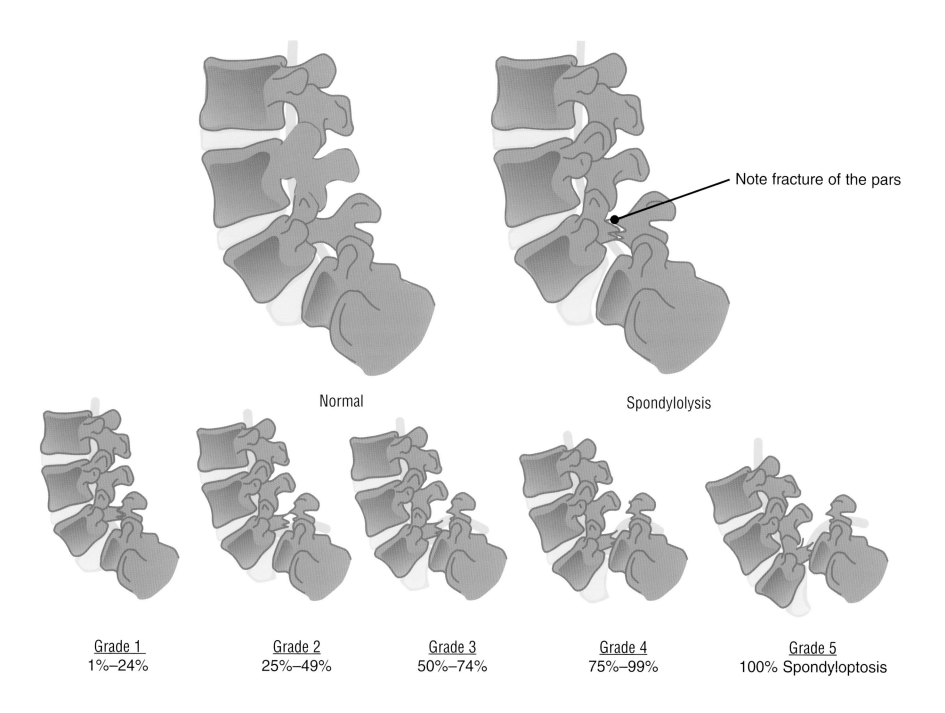

Note fracture of the pars

Normal

Spondylolysis

Grade 1
1%–24%

Grade 2
25%–49%

Grade 3
50%–74%

Grade 4
75%–99%

Grade 5
100% Spondyloptosis

Scoliosis

Scoliosis is a condition in which the vertebral bodies are rotated, creating various prominences. The cause of scoliosis cannot commonly be found. The majority of cases are called idiopathic, usually found in adolescent girls.

Exercise, lifting, sports, posture and small leg length discrepancies do not cause scoliosis.

Classically, scoliosis is painless. However, when pain is present, it consists of back pain and a dull pain progressing distally from the buttock into the leg in a specific zone. A historical evaluation of the patient's birth, delivery and development may help to assess if there is a neuromuscular or congenital abnormality. There may be a family history of scoliosis.

Physical examination is carried in the Adam's forward bend position with arms extended and knees straight. The examiner assesses for prominences in the thorax or the lower trunk. A full neurological assessment is necessary.

Brace treatment (orthosis) is typically recommended in children with spinal deformity and curve magnitudes of 25 to 40 degrees. Brace treatment is recommended only in children with remaining potential to grow (i.e., the skeleton is immature).

Surgical treatments include posterior spinal fusion, instrumentation and bone grafting. At times anterior surgical stabilization may be recommended. With modern-day techniques, patients are rapidly ambulatory and usually discharged from the hospital within 5–7 days after surgery. Postoperative casting and bracing are not required in most cases.

Normal Spine   Scoliosis-Curved Spine

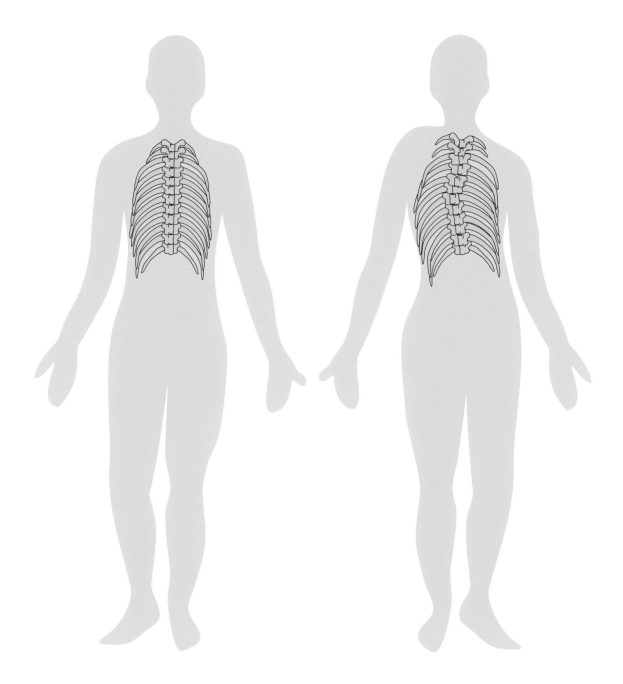

Medical Evaluations of the Patient for Spine Surgery

Basic Medical Evaluation
Vascular Evaluation
Cardiac Evaluation
Hematological Evaluation

Basic Medical Evaluation

Before proceeding with spinal surgery, patients are recommended to have an evaluation by a medical doctor for general medical clearance. Specific attention is paid to the heart, lungs, arteries, brain and spinal system. The medical physician evaluates the entire patient with special regard for any potential problems that may develop at or around the time of surgery.

Comorbidity Weighted Index	
Assigned Weights for Disease	Disease
1	• Myocardial Infarct • Congestive Heart Failure • Peripheral Vascular Diseas • Cerebrovascular Accident • Dementia • Chronic Pulmonary Disease • Connective Tissue Disease • Gastrointestinal Ulcer Disease • Mild Liver Disease • Diabetes Mellitus
2	• Hemiplegia • Moderate to Severe Renal Disease • Diabetes with End Organ Damage • Any Tumor • Leukemia • Lymphoma
3	• Moderate or Severe Liver Disease
6	• Autoimmune Deficiency Syndrome • Metastatic Solid Tumor

Reproduced with permission of Clinical Orthopedics & Related Research.

Vascular Evaluation

A complete evaluation before surgery includes an evaluation of the arteries and veins. For example, a patient with an aortic or carotid aneurysm may not be an ideal candiate for hypotensive anesthesia.

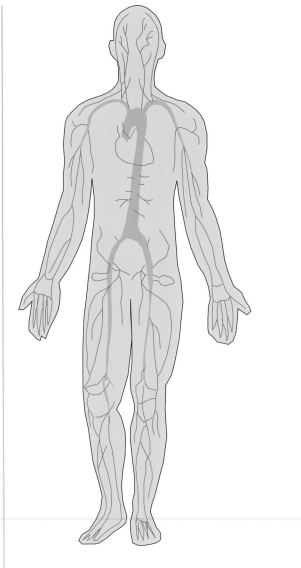

Cardiac Evaluation

Cardiac events continue to be the leading cause of suffering after major surgeries. Dr. Thomas Faciszewski and colleagues made specific recommendations for the evaluation of the patient with lumbar spinal stenosis. These protocols are defined to the right.

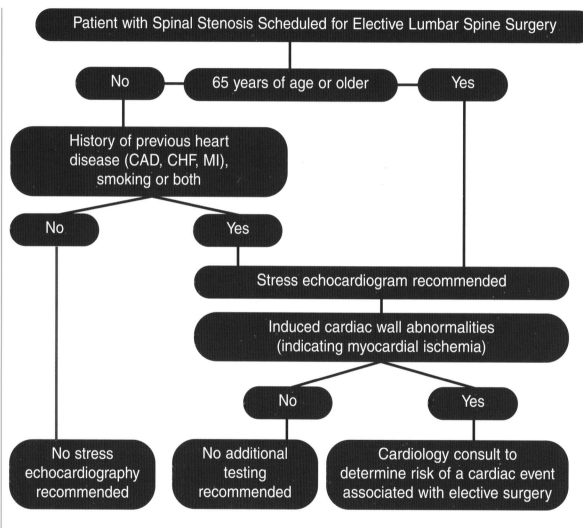

Reproduced with permission of Clinical Orthopedics & Related Research.

Cardiac Evaluation

The factors associated with the risk of having a heart problem during surgery have been defined.

Predictors of Perioperative Myocardial Infarction		
Major	Intermediate	Minor
• Recent myocardial infarction with continued ischemia • Unstable angina • Decompensated congestive heart failure • Severe valvular disease • Significant arrhythmias	• Mild angina • Prior myocardial infarction • Compensated congestive heart failure • Diabetes mellitus	• Advanced age • Abnormal electrocardiogram • Nonsinus cardiac rhythms • Low functional capacity

Reproduced with permission of Clinical Orthopedics & Related Research.

Hematological Evaluation

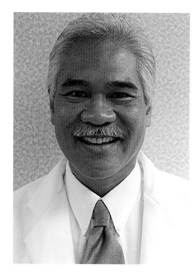

Edgar M. Alvarez, M.D.

The hematologist evaluates the patient for bleeding problems. This physician's sole concern is the assessment of the patient's blood parameters. In certain cases, the hematologist may recommend various interventions, including vitamins, food supplements, or medications. In the hospital, the hematologist follows up on the patient after surgery and makes further recommendations.

For example, in one of Jehovah's Witnesses, erythropoietin may be recommended to increase the blood levels before surgery but it would be up to the individual Witness to accept or refrain.

In a hemophiliac, the diagnosis may be confirmed by testing, and specific factors recommended before, during, and after surgery.

Hematological Evaluation

Considerations for treatment with epoetin alfa have been defined in accordance to the recommendations of Dr. E. Michael Keating.

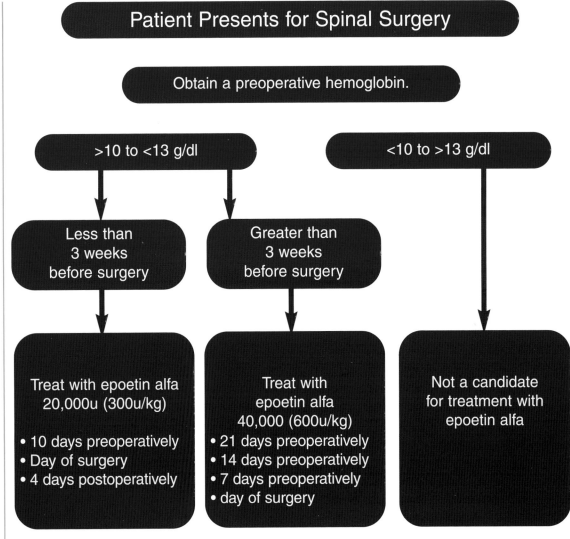

Patient Presents for Spinal Surgery

Obtain a preoperative hemoglobin.

>10 to <13 g/dl

<10 to >13 g/dl

Less than 3 weeks before surgery

Greater than 3 weeks before surgery

Treat with epoetin alfa 20,000u (300u/kg)
- 10 days preoperatively
- Day of surgery
- 4 days postoperatively

Treat with epoetin alfa 40,000 (600u/kg)
- 21 days preoperatively
- 14 days preoperatively
- 7 days preoperatively
- day of surgery

Not a candidate for treatment with epoetin alfa

An important concern to be addressed, at least a month before surgery when feasible, is the patient's levels of hemoglobin and iron. Occasionally, if the physician suspects severe anemia or nutritional deficiencies, he or she will order other tests such as a reticulocyte count or folate and vitamin B12 levels.

The most important thing patients can do to prepare for the surgery is to take care of themselves physically and to eat as healthily as possible. Even if the patient is vegetarian, there are foods that can improve the body's iron storage. Iron is important because it is the component of hemoglobin that delivers oxygen to the tissues. Iron is also essential for a red blood cell development. In addition, in patients who are anemic and may need a drug called erythropoietin, iron plays a vital role as a supplement.

A coordinator will discuss the results of the patient's blood work. This information goes to the surgeon and anesthesiologist as well. If the patient is only slightly anemic, the coordinator may recommend oral iron and vitamins.

A typical regimen includes:

- 65 mg of elemental iron (ferrous sulfate 325 mg) by mouth three times a day. Iron is much better absorbed on an empty stomach, but may be less well tolerated that way.

- Folic acid 1 mg orally once a day. This promotes normal red blood cell formation and enhances the work of the iron.

- Vitamin C 500 mg per day. Vitamin C (ascorbic acid) helps form and maintain tissues and capillary walls.

If the patient's hemoglobin level is between 10 and 13 g/dL, and he or she is scheduled for elective, noncardiac, nonvascular surgeries, the patient falls into a small category of patients for whom the doctor may choose to use a drug called erythropoietin alfa to boost red blood cell production. This drug is given in once weekly injections and is very effective when used with iron supplements.

The coordinator can explore the reimbursement issues pertaining to this drug as well. Negotiation with the insurer may be required, another reason for expressing the patient's wish for transfusion-free surgery as early as possible.

If the patient's hemoglobin falls below 10, and there is a potential for significant blood loss, the responsible party may choose to refer the patient to a hematologist to ensure the best possible surgical outcome.

Preoperative Bloodless Assessments for Jehovah's Witness

In the case of Jehovah's Witnesses, the coordinator is there to clarify the patient's wishes regarding transfusions. The coordinator will ask the patient for advanced medical directives and a health proxy, and go over the "conscience categories." With the advancement in understanding of molecular biology and how blood works, the Watchtower Society has recognized that certain fractions of blood pass the placental barrier. *Three Questions from Readers in The Watchtower* may be helpful in making decisions. They can be found in the June 1, 1990, and the June 15 and October 15, 2000 issues. Today many of Jehovah's Witnesses will choose to accept these conscience categories, including albumin and clotting factors. This issue is important to discuss and clarify as drugs like erythropoietin contain a small drop of albumin. The use of special closed circuits for cell salvage for Jehovah's Witnesses make this process acceptable to most, but its use should be discussed.

The coordinator is there as part of the team, helping to facilitate patient's care. She or he will monitor patient's postoperative progress daily, with special attention to the frequency of laboratory draws and the results of blood work. The coordinator will make sure that the correct wrist band is on the patient and an over-bed sign is posted, notifying everybody who cares for the patient that he or she does not wish blood transfusions.

If the patient is a minor (under the age of 18) and is not emancipated, the law requires that, if the life is in jeopardy doctors must take whatever measures are necessary to try to save the patient. However, a bloodless surgery program is designed to ensure that all possible nonblood alternatives will be explored first.

Spine Surgery

Intraoperative Monitoring
Surgical Instruments
Surgical Procedures

Radial Arterial Catheter

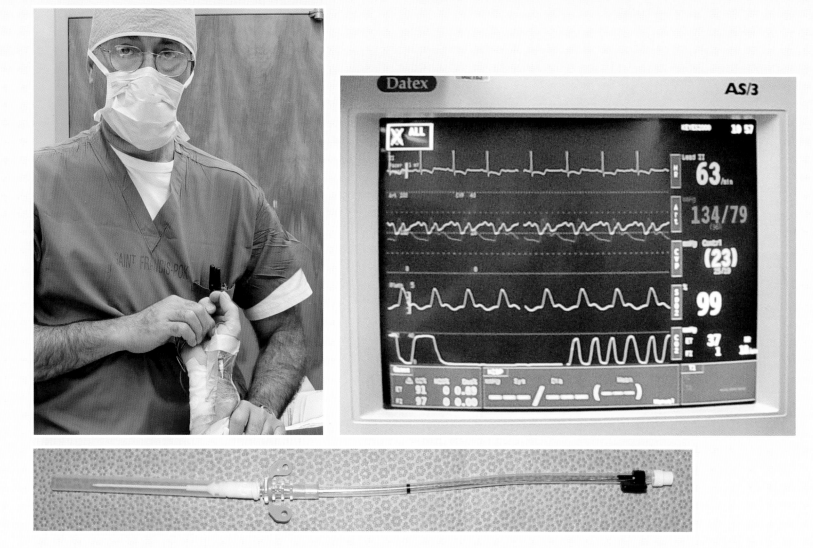

A radial arterial catheter may be used to assess the patient's blood pressure directly and accurately.

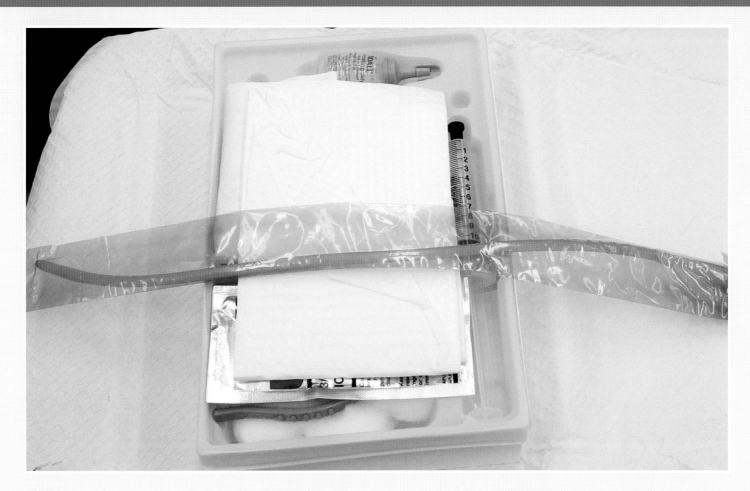

A foley catheter may be used to measure urine output, an important factor in fluid performance of the body.

Central Access Catheter

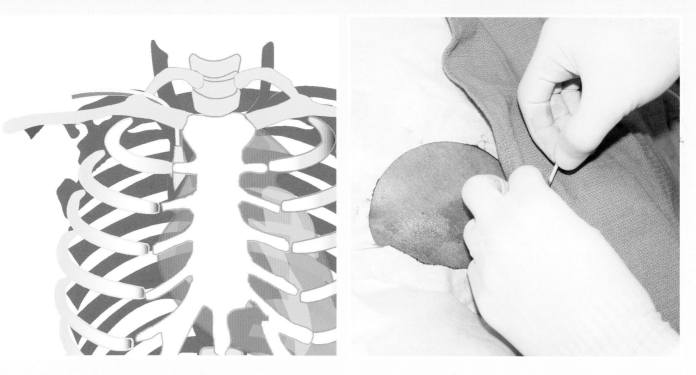

Over the past 25 years, the clinical use of central vein catheters has increased with medical and technological advances, especially in emergency resuscitation protocols and sophisticated monitoring techniques. Expeditious placement of central intravenous catheters is necessary when there are large fluid shifts, especially with consideration for hypotensive anesthesia. Fortunately, large veins (such as the subclavican vein and internal jugular vein) have constant, predictable relationships to easily identifiable anatomic landmarks.

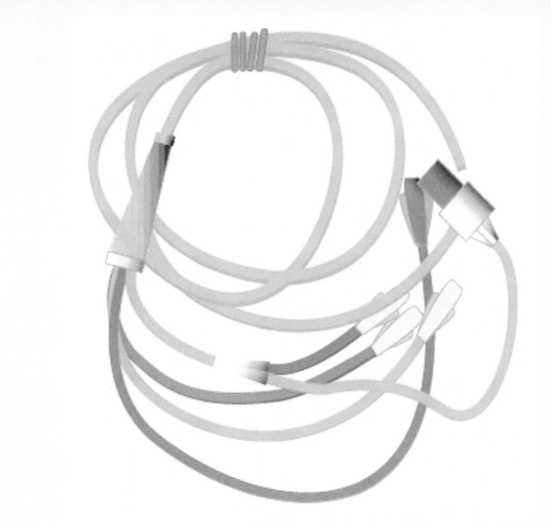

The utilization of the balloon-flotation, flow-directed pulmonary artery thermodilution Swan-Ganz catheter perhaps best symbolizes modern care of the critically ill patient.

Regional Anesthesia

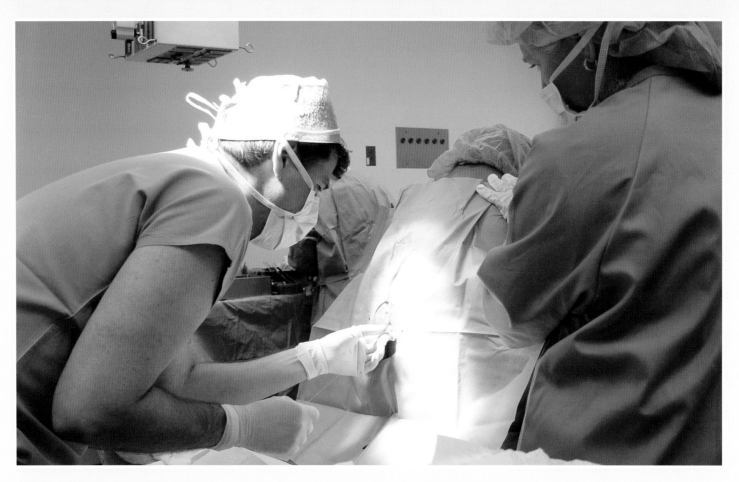

The anesthesiologist, at times, may choose to apply regional anesthesia techniques, which may further help to diminish blood loss.

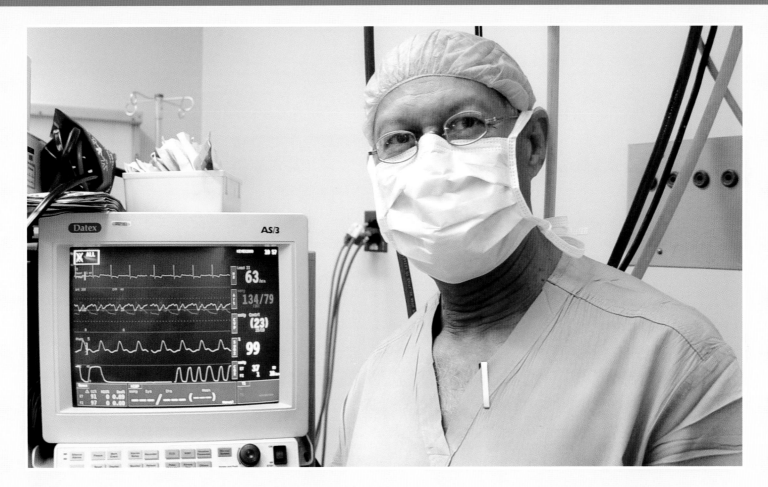

With careful clinical judgment, the anesthesiologist may lower the patient's blood pressure in surgery, further reducing blood loss. The anesthesiologist may send blood samples to the lab to monitor blood levels and electrolytes.

Fluroscopic Evaluation

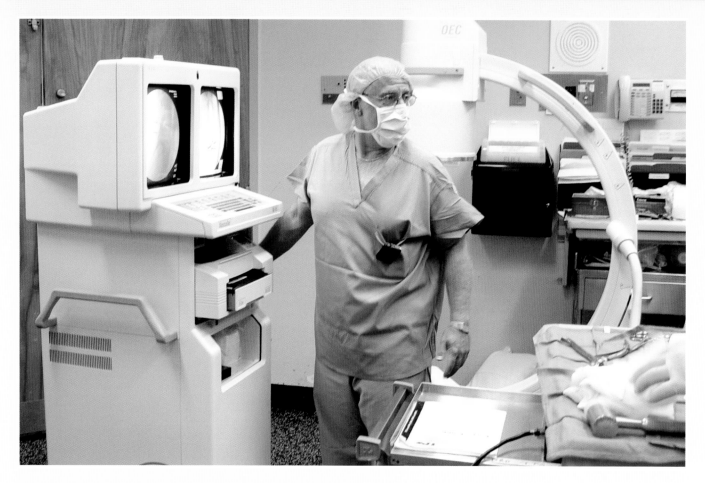

During surgery, the fluroscope may be used to precisely pinpoint the area to be operated on. This leads to less dissection and blood loss.

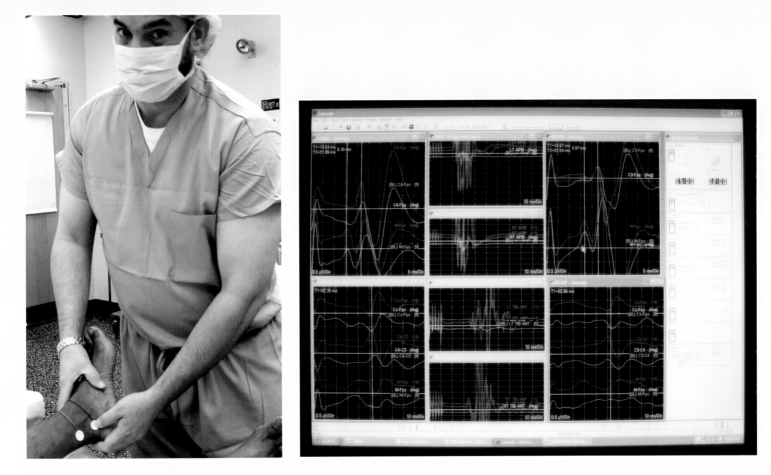

A neuromonitoring specialist may attach leads to the body. The leads monitor the muscles for nerve and spinal cord activity. During surgery, any motion or activity of the nerve root is noted on the monitor by depolarization. Audible monitors are also used. Neuromonitoring increases the safety of performing spinal surgery.

Considerations of Lumbar Spinal Stenosis

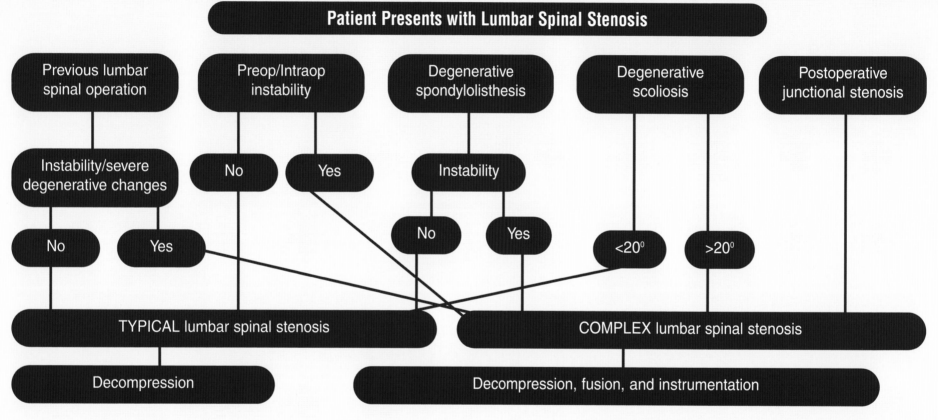

Reproduced with permission of Clinical Orthopedics & Related Research.

Decisions for the surgery are complicated. Making decisions before the operation leads to more precision, less exploring, and diminished blood loss.

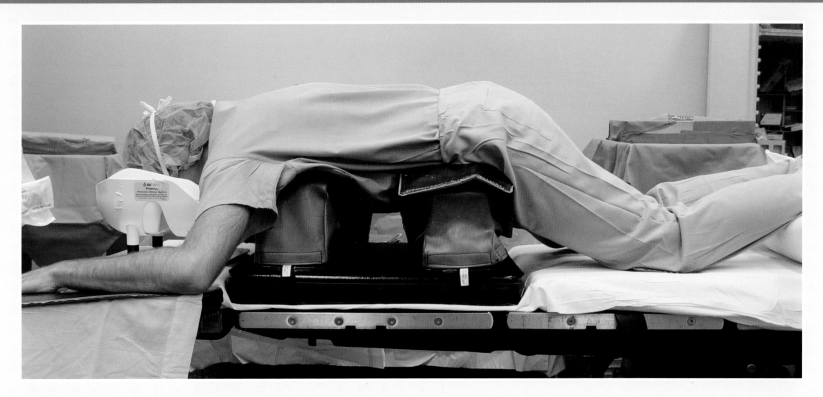

In the operating room, the patient is placed on a four poster table. The four posters supports the iliac crests (pelvis) and the chest wall. Note that the abdomen is allowed to hang freely. When the abdomen is free, the great vessels (aorta and vena cava) are in a dependent position. The pooling of blood in the dependent position leads to significantly less blood loss.

Bovie Coagulator and Bipolar Coagulator

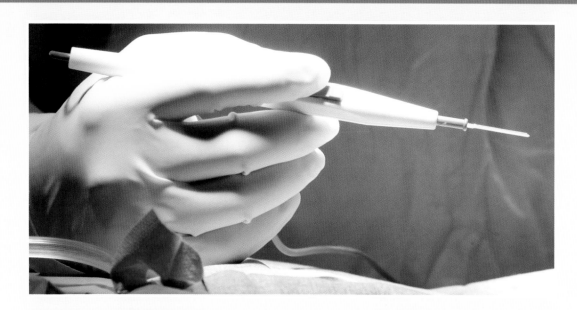

The Bovie coagulator (also known as monopolar) allows coagulation by sending electricity from the tip of the instrument to a grounding pad (usually on the leg).

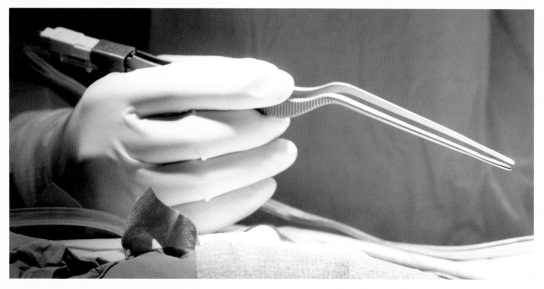

The bipolar coagulator allows the surgeon to coagulate between the tips of a fine instrument, preventing electrical current from traveling to the rest of the body. This device is used near the spinal cord and nerve roots.

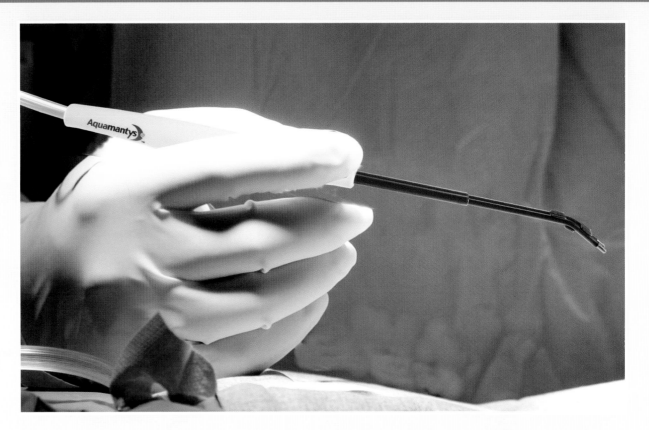

The Aquamantys™ System is designed to seal blood vessels in soft tissue and bone with a significant potential to diminish intra-operative blood loss, and therefore post-operative transfusion. This system uses bipolar radiofrequency energy simultaneously cooled with saline water solution to stop bleeding by sealing blood vessels. Saline water solution keeps the process at a relatively low temperature of 60 – 100° C.

Harmonic Scalpel

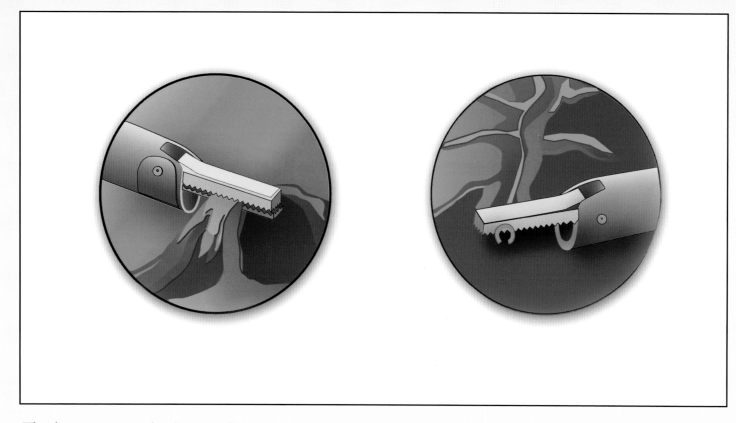

The harmonic scalpel uses ultrasonic energy to cut and coagulate soft tissue. Because no electricity passes to or through the patient, the potential hazards of monopolar surgery are eliminated. Precise cutting with minimal lateral thermal tissue damage allows the harmonic scalpel to be used for dissection near vital structures.

High-Intensity Headlights

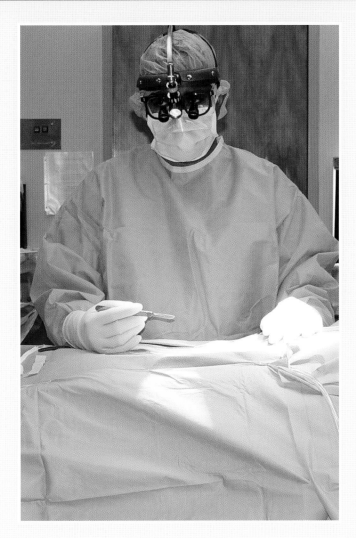

The surgical field is better observed with high-intensity headlights. Better vision means less blood loss. (A traditional surgical knife is shown here.) Magnified vision is provided with the use of loupes (shown here). Other times microscopes are used in surgery.

Futuristic Surgical Suite

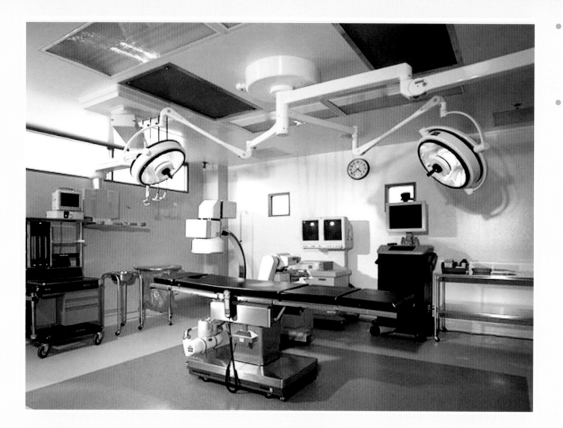

- A complete digital television station provides global connectivity and cyber-teleconferencing capability.

- Advanced surgical equipment:
    - Surgical robotics
    - Laser machines
    - Image guided surgical system
    - Radio frequency instrument
    - Neurophysiological monitors
    - Digital image enhanced endoscopy

Dr. John Chiu of the California Spine Center presents the edge of development of minimally invasive techniques and instrumentation.

Innovative "Bloodless" Instruments

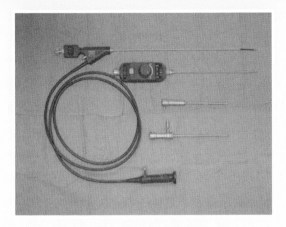

Steerable Spinoscope

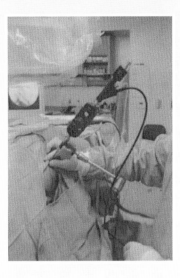

Endoscope in Surgery

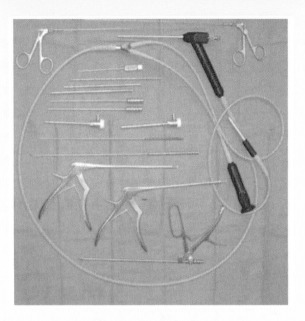

Cervicothoracoscope

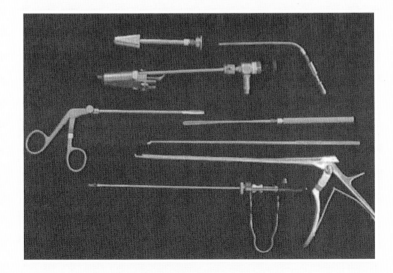

Endospine System

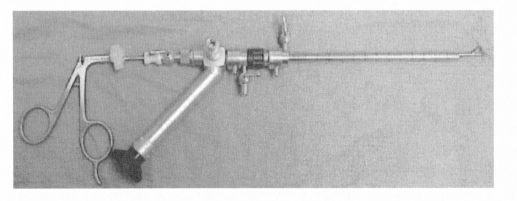

Lumbar Foraminascope

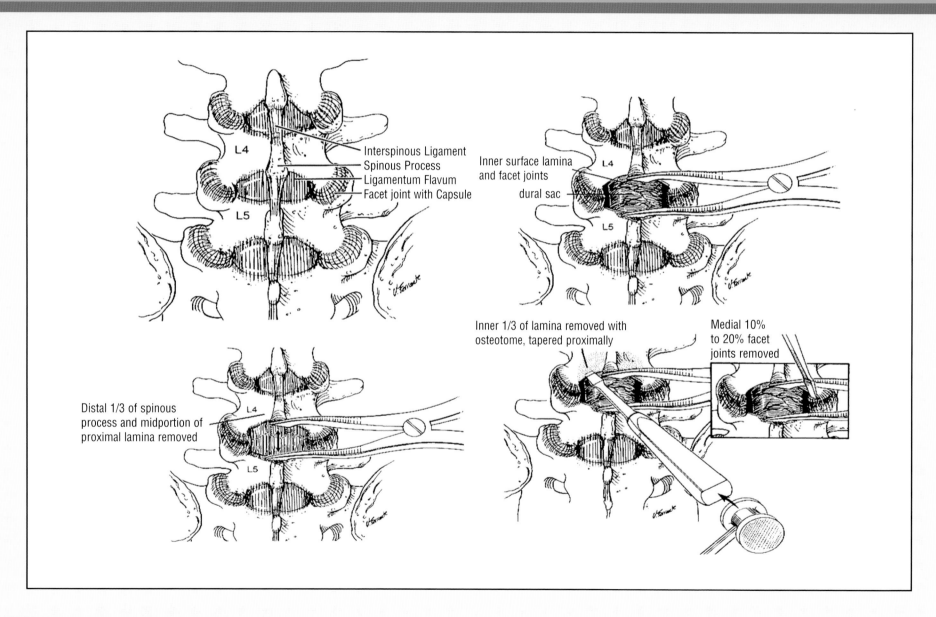

L4

L5

Interspinous Ligament
Spinous Process
Ligamentum Flavum
Facet joint with Capsule

Inner surface lamina
and facet joints

dural sac

L4

L5

Distal 1/3 of spinous
process and midportion of
proximal lamina removed

Inner 1/3 of lamina removed with
osteotome, tapered proximally

Medial 10%
to 20% facet
joints removed

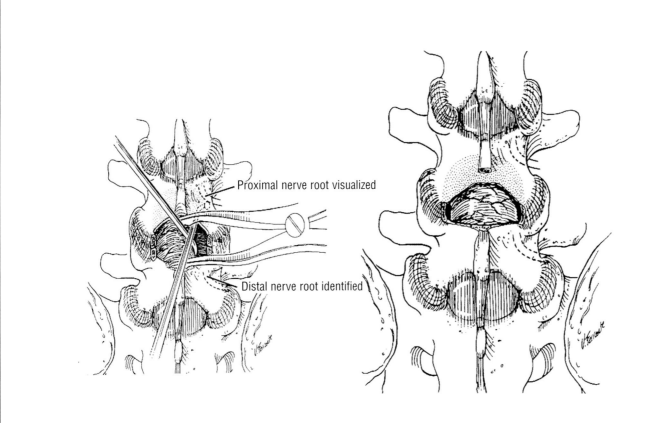

Proximal nerve root visualized

Distal nerve root identified

Dr. Patrick F. O'Leary described his technique of distraction laminaplasty. This procedure resects much less bone, while still allowing for decompression of the spinal sac and nerve roots by distraction. This translates to less blood loss and increases postoperative stability of the spine.

Reproduced with permission of CORR.

Minimally Invasive Techniques for Discectomy

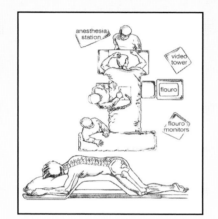

Typical operating room set-up

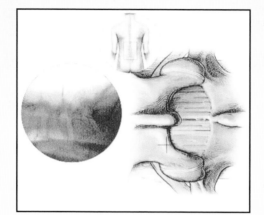

X-ray and anatomical alignment

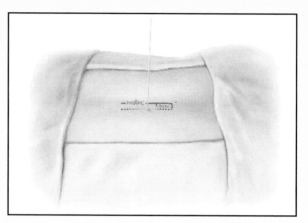

Guide wire precisely placed

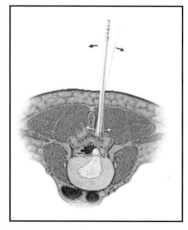

Initial dilators placed

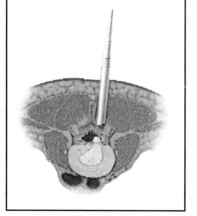

Sequential dilators placed

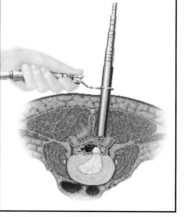

Tubular retractor inserted

With modern-day minimally invasive techniques, surgeons make precise placements of smaller incisions, do less dissection of muscles, and at times do operations through tubes. This leads to less blood loss on the table, less possible complications, faster recovery and speedier return to work time.

Reproduced with permission of Sofamor Danek.

Minimally Invasive Techniques for Discectomy

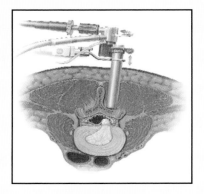

Endoscope Inserted with

Light Source

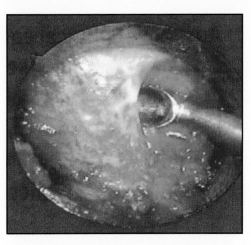

Lamina and LigamentumFlavum

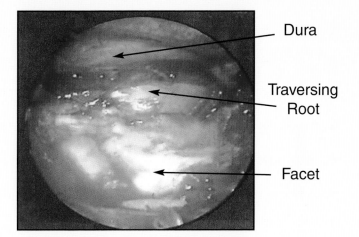

Dura

Traversing
Root

Facet

Nerve Root Isolated

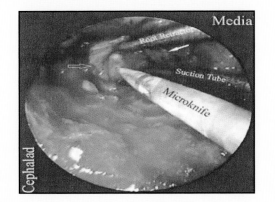

Media

Root Retractor

Suction Tube

Microknife

Cephalad

Annulus Incised

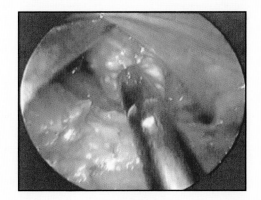

Disc Removed

Kyphoplasty

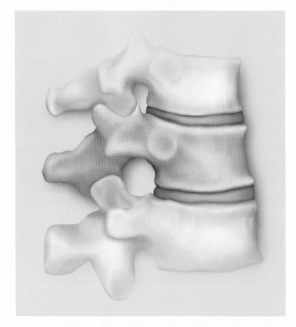

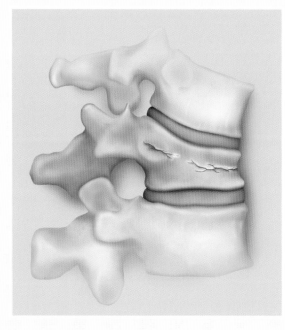

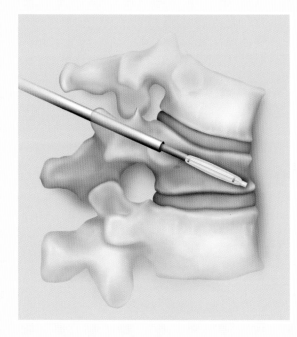

1. Normal Vertebra

2. Fractured Vertebra

Vertebra Body Compression
Fracture

3. Precise Access

Through a small incision, the
doctor creates a narrow pathway
into the fractured bone.

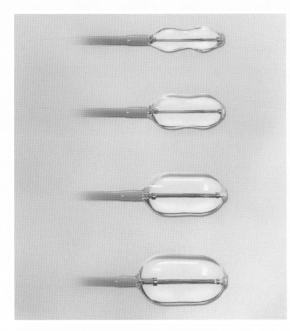

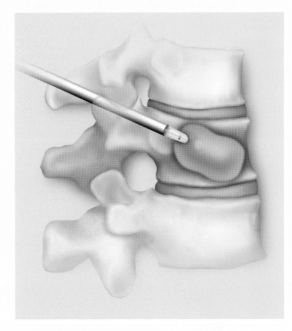

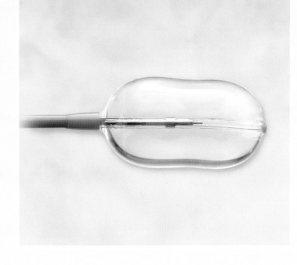

4. Balloon Inflated

The balloon is inflated, moving the collapsed portion of the vertebra. The purpose is to restore the fractured bone to its original shape.

5. Balloon Removal

Once the doctor has achieved the desired result, the balloon is deflated and removed. The doctor can then finish the procedure.

6. Cement Placed

Cement is then placed in the cavity.

Reproduced with permission of Kyphon.

Vitagel

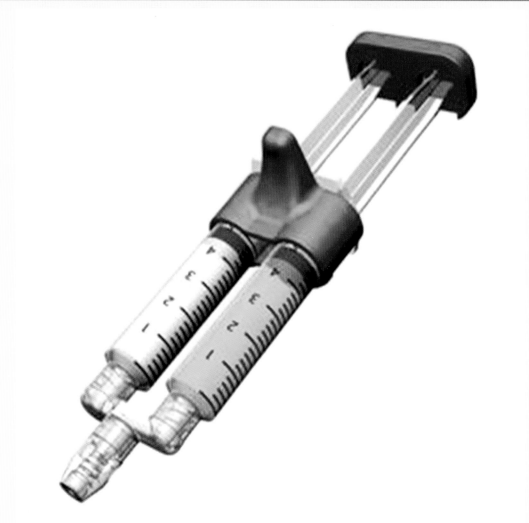

Vitagel™ is an FDA approved surgical hemostat used to control bleeding and facilitate healing while utilizing the patient's own biology. Vitagel™ is composed of microfibrillar collagen and thrombin in combination with the patient's own plasma which contains fibrinogen and platelets. This unique combination of components produces an effective and safe hemostat by forming a collagen/fibrin scaffold with platelets.

Patient Case Reports

Standard Spine Decompression
Complex Spine Reconstruction
Spinal Fusion-Jehovah's Witness
Spinal Fusion-Hemophilia
Kyphoplasty

Standard Spine Decompression

Thomas L. was treated with a standard discectomy and osteophytectomy.

Spinal decompression procedures serve to relieve pressure from nerve roots and the spinal canal. These procedures are common.

- Blood loss was minimal in surgery.

- Cell saver was not used because of minimal blood loss.

- Autologous donation was not recommended because of minimal blood loss.

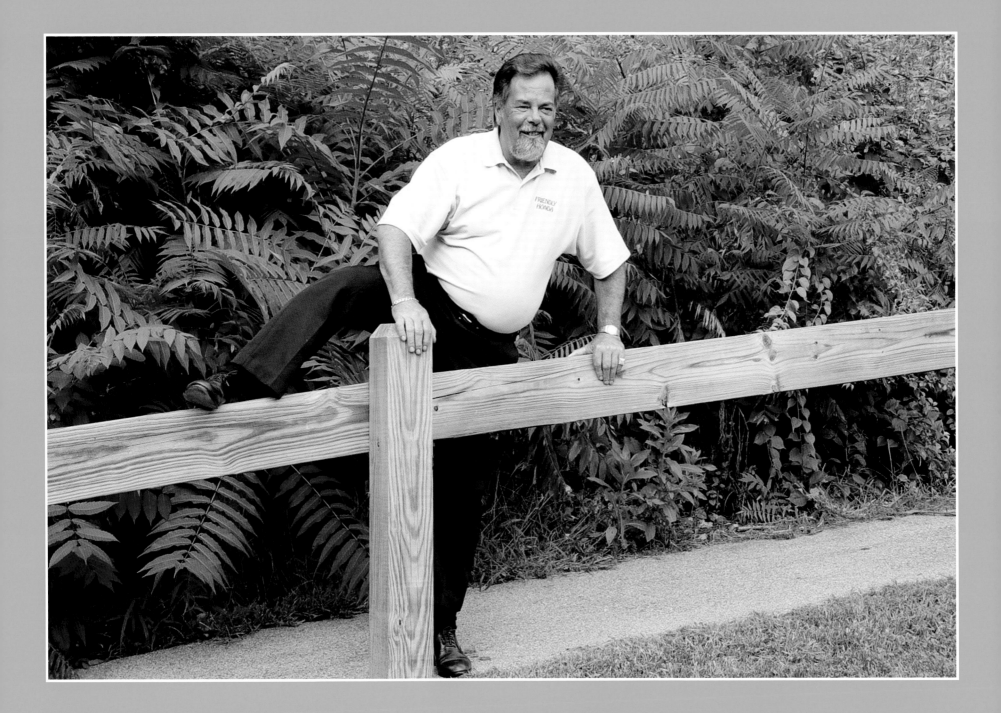

Complex Spine Reconstruction

Marlene M. was treated with anterior and posterior spinal fusion previously. She was evaluated and found to have junctional breakdown with lumbar spinal stenosis and discogenic disease.

Spinal fusion surgeries are more complicated than decompressive surgeries. Usually adjacent segments are stabilized with the use of instruments and bone graft.

- Marlene underwent a successful reconstruction of the previous fusion with extension (anteriorly and posteriorly) to the junctional level.

- Blood loss was minimal in surgery.

- Cell saver was used in surgery.

- Autologous donation of blood was utilized.

- The patient received only her own blood back.

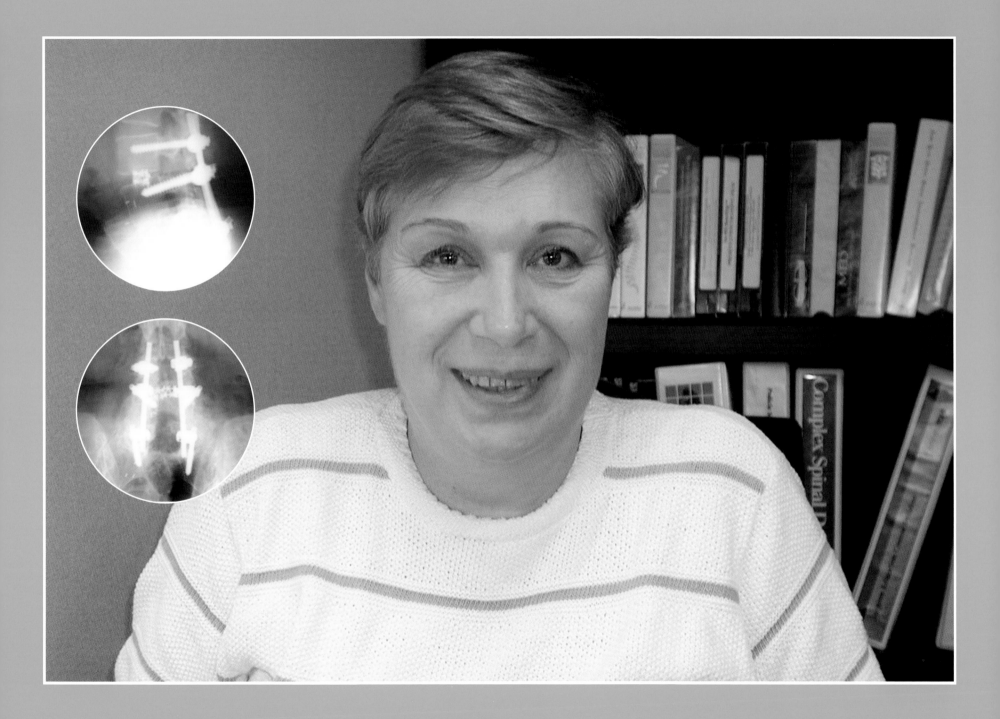

Spinal Fusion—Jehovah's Witnessess

Luis R. underwent spinal fusion surgery. The patient chose not to accept any blood product, including autotransfusion with his own blood during surgery.

It is estimated that there are more than 2 million Jehovah's Witnesses in the United States.

Followers of this religion believe that the Bible prohibits blood or blood product transfusion (Acts 15:28–29). Typically, patients of this religion do not accept transfusions of whole blood, packed cells, white blood cells, platelets, plasma or autotransfusion of predeposited blood.

Some Witnesses may permit infusion of albumin, clotting factor solutions, or dextran or other plasma expanders and intraoperative autotransfusion, done under closed loop technique.

Even though a transfusion may be necessary to save a patient's life, the administration of blood and/or blood products in the face of refusal after informed consent can be legally considered a violation of a patient's right to control what is done to his or her body.

In the awake, fully informed and otherwise competent adult patient has decided against transfusion, courts have ruled that physicians cannot be held liable if they comply with that patient's directive and withhold life-saving blood administration due to specific and detailed consent.

The issue becomes difficult when patients are unconscious (most Jehovah's Witnesses carry cards informing medical personnel of their religious beliefs) or minors.

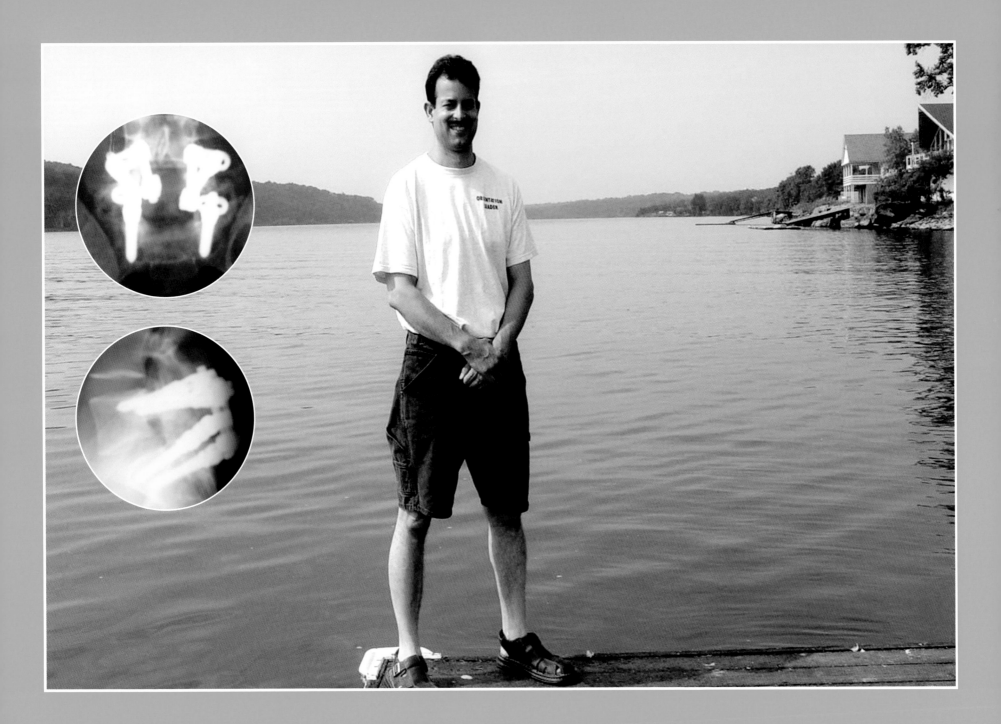

Spinal Fusion—Hemophilia

Frank D. underwent safe spinal fusion surgery for a painful spondylolyis defect.

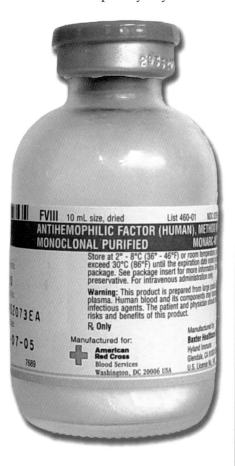

Hemophilia is a disease of missing or insufficient bleeding factors.

Classic hemophilia is caused by Factor VIII deficiency, while hemophilia A and Christmas disease are caused by Factor IX deficiency.

Surgical treatment of hemophilia, hemophilia A, hemophilia B, and Christmas disease have become possible and reasonable with the availability of Factor VIII and Factor IX concentrates. The cost of factor treatment is high.

Previously, only lifesaving surgery was performed, and the death rate was high. Wound bleeding with massive sloughs and infection were common. However, only by expert management and strict control of the clotting mechanism can serious complications be minimized, and therefore surgery in patients with hemophilia must not be undertaken casually.

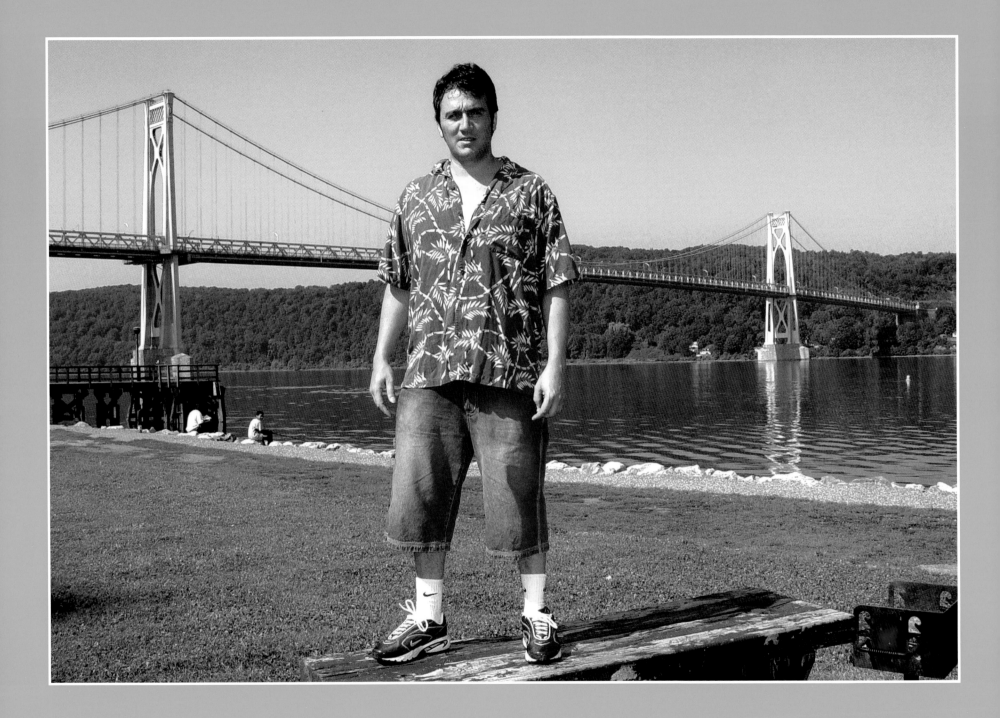

Osteoporosis

Elena J. underwent kyphoplasty
surgery successfully.

Osteoporosis, or porous bone, is a disease characterized by low bone mass and structural deterioration of bone tissue, leading to bone fragility and an increased susceptibility to fractures of the hip, spine and wrist.

The National Osteoporosis Foundation estimates that osteoporosis is a major public health threat for 44 million Americans (80 percent of whom are women). Of that total, 10 million are estimated to already have the disease and nearly 34 million are estimated to have low bone mass, placing them at an increased risk for osteoporosis.

Osteoporosis is responsible for more than 1.5 million fractures annually. Osteoporosis is often called the "silent disease" because bone loss occurs without symptoms. People may not know they have osteoporosis until their bones become so weak that a sudden strain, bump, or fall causes a fracture or a vertebra to collapse. Collapsed vertebrae may initially be felt or seen in the form of severe back pain, loss of height or spinal deformities such as kyphosis (stooped posture).

While early diagnosis and treatment provide the best options for patients with osteoporosis, current treatment options approved by the U.S. Food and Drug Administration (FDA) for the prevention and treatment of postmenopausal osteoporosis include estrogen and progesterone hormone replacement therapy, alendronate, risedronate, bisphosphonates, raloxifene, selective estrogen receptor modulator, and recombinant parathyroid hormone. Calcitonin is approved for treatment only.

Additional treatment options include limited bed rest, braces and, in the case of a broken bone, fracture reduction and fixation to facilitate healing.

Recently, fracture reduction and fixation with polymethylmethacrylete became available.

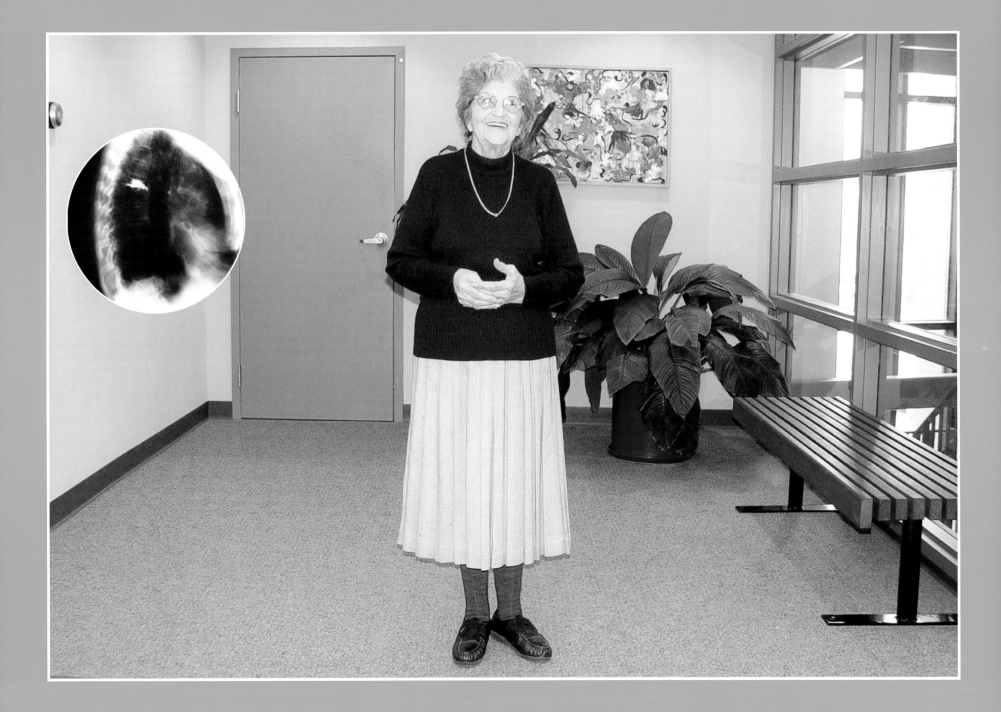

Dictionary of Bloodless Terminology

Acute Normovolemic Hemodilution

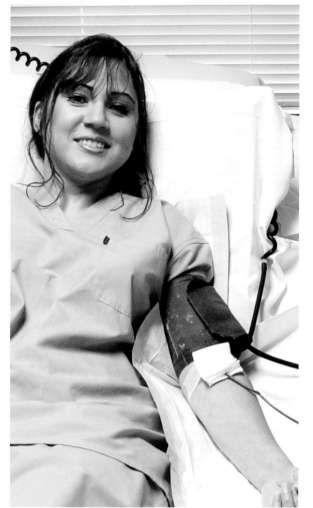

Patient:

The process of collecting blood from the patient and replacing it with substitute fluids in order to reduce the amount of "actual blood" the patient bleeds. The anesthesiologist determines, based on the patient's cardiac and pulmonary condition, if the patient is able to tolerate the removal of blood from the body prior to surgery. If so, blood is then withdrawn from a vein through a tube that stays connected to the patient's blood system during surgery; the anesthesiologist then replaces the extracted volume with the substitute fluids. Therefore, when the patient bleeds, he or she is losing the substitute fluids and much less of his or her own vital blood. When it is time to re-infuse, the blood is allowed to return to the body.

Clinical:

Intraoperative hemodilution removes 1 to 3 units of the patient's blood and replaces it with crystalloid or, in some cases, a combination of crystalloid and colloid to restore the intravascular volume. This is done before an operation and is tolerated well in all patient populations. The blood that is withdrawn is anticoagulated and maintained at room temperature for up to 4 hours. It is re-infused into the patient as needed during the surgical procedure. If this procedure is combined with autologous donation prior to surgery, 6 or more units of blood can be available for a procedure in which significant blood loss is expected.

Murray D. Acute normovolemic hemodilution. Eur Spine J. 2004 Oct;13 Suppl 1:S72-5.

Loubser PG, Chan A. Prediction of the effect of acute normovolemic hemodilution on the hematological constituents of sequestered autologous whole blood. Anesth Analg. 2006 Apr;102(4):991-7.

Monk TG. Acute normovolemic hemodilution. Anesthesiol Clin North America. 2005 Jun;23(2):271-81,

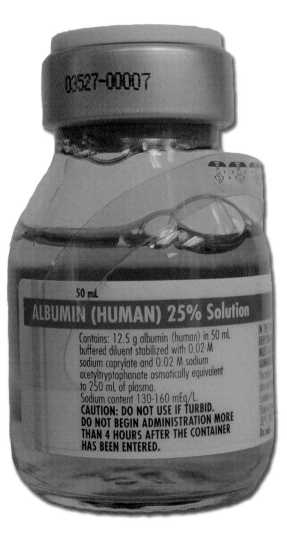

ALBUMIN (HUMAN) 25% Solution

Contains: 12.5 g albumin (human) in 50 mL buffered diluent stabilized with 0.02 M sodium caprylate and 0.02 M sodium acetyltryptophanate osmotically equivalent to 250 mL of plasma.
Sodium content 130-160 mEq/L.
CAUTION: DO NOT USE IF TURBID.
DO NOT BEGIN ADMINISTRATION MORE THAN 4 HOURS AFTER THE CONTAINER HAS BEEN ENTERED.

Patient:

A fraction of blood that is used to regulate the volume of circulating blood. When it is administered in a low concentration, it works like normal human plasma. When it is administered in a higher concentration, it helps to draw fluid from the patient's body into his or her arteries and veins. Albumin may be acceptable to some patients who refuse blood for religious reasons.

Clinical:

This product is derived from donated blood collected by the American Red Cross Blood Services. Albumin is a highly soluble ellipsoidal protein (MW: 66,500) accounting for 70–80% of the colloid osmotic pressure of plasma. Albumin is very important in regulating the volume of circulating blood. When injected intravenously, 5% albumin will increase the circulating plasma volume by an amount approximately equal to the volume infused. Twenty-five percent albumin, when injected intravenously, will draw approximately 3.5 times its volume of additional fluid into the circulation within 15 minutes.

Adams HA, Piepenbrock S, Hempelmann G. Volume replacement solutions—pharmacology and clinical use. Anasthesiol Intensivmed Notfallmed Schmerzther. 1998 Jan;33(1):2-17.

Allogenic Blood

Blood that is donated to the blood bank by a volunteer and used by a patient in need. Usually donated blood is split into parts, such as packed red cells, plasma, platelets, or certain white cell preparations. Today, blood is considered safer than it has ever been. Many countries have included in their processing of donated blood a treatment, known as leukocyte reduction, that decreases the likelihood of immune suppression (one of the most significant side effects of receiving several or more units of blood). Jehovah's Witnesses believe, in their interpretation of scripture, that the transfusion of blood and its major components is unacceptable. For this reason, bloodless surgery is not just an alternative for these patients but an absolute necessity.

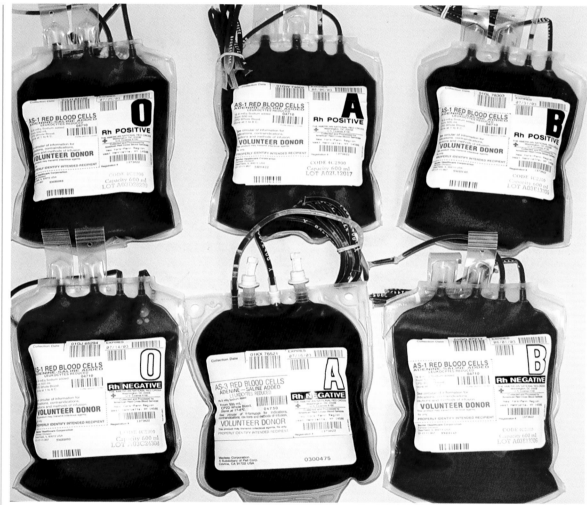

Moore EE, Johnson JL, Cheng AM, Masuno T, Banerjee A. Insights from studies of blood substitutes in trauma. Shock. 2005 Sep;24(3):197-205.

Blood donors are healthy volunteers typically over the age of 17, at least 110 pounds in weight, and are screened through a detailed medical history. Once donated, the blood is processed into its various parts such as red blood cells, platelets, and plasma.

Approximately 70% of the blood products are filtered to remove leukocytes (white blood cells) that fight foreign elements such as bacteria, viruses and abnormal cells that may cause disease. When leukocytes are present in donated blood, they may not be tolerated by the person receiving the blood and cause transfusion complications.

The various blood components are labeled according to blood type and Rh factor (O+, A+, B+, AB+, O–, A–, B–, AB–).

Transfusion Risk

- Antibodies to HIV-1 and HIV-2 (AIDS)

- Antibodies to HBc produced during and after infection with Hepatitis B virus

- Antibodies to HCV produced after infection with the Hepatitis C virus

- Antibodies to HTLV-I/II produced after infection with Human T-lym photropic virus (HTLV-I and HTLV-II)

- Antibodies to HBsAg produced after infection with hepatitis B

- For blood type (ABO) and Rh factor

- Tp (the agent that causes syphilis)

- Liver enzyme ALT (An elevated ALT may indicate liver inflammation, which may be caused by a hepatitis virus)

- The presence of unexpected antibodies that may cause reactions after the transfusion

- CMV (a test for the cytomegalovirus—performed on physician request)

- NAT (nucleic acid testing, a new technology that can detect the genetic material of hepatitis C and HIV)

Ellis FR, Friedman LI, Wirak BF, Hellinger MJ, Malin WS, Greenwalt TJ. A computerized national Blood Donor Deferral Register. JAMA. 1975 May 19;232(7):722-4.

Allogenic Blood—Risks of Transfusion

Transfusion	Risk
HIV	1 /1 ,000,000
Hepatitis B	1/100,000
Hepatitis C	1/500—1/500,000
HTLV I and II	1/200,000
Bacterial sepsis—platelets	1/10,000
Bacterial sepsis—red cells	Less Than 1/1,000,000
Hemolytic reactions—acute	1 in 24,000; fatal 1 in 600,000
Hemolytic reactions—delayed	1 in 2,500; fatal 1 in 6,000

Though blood is collected from healthy volunteer donors and is tested for a variety of disease causing viruses, there are still risks. Presently, the greatest risk for an infectious transfusion is bacterial contamination from the handling and storage of collected units.

Pomper GJ, Wu Y, Snyder EL. Risks of transfusion-transmitted infections: 2003. Curr Opin Hematol. 2003 Nov;10(6):412-8.

Patient:

Antibodies are used by the body to identify what is "foreign." After foreign material is identified, it may be targeted for destruction.

Clinical:

The response of the body, using antibodies, when exposed to foreign substances such as antigens.

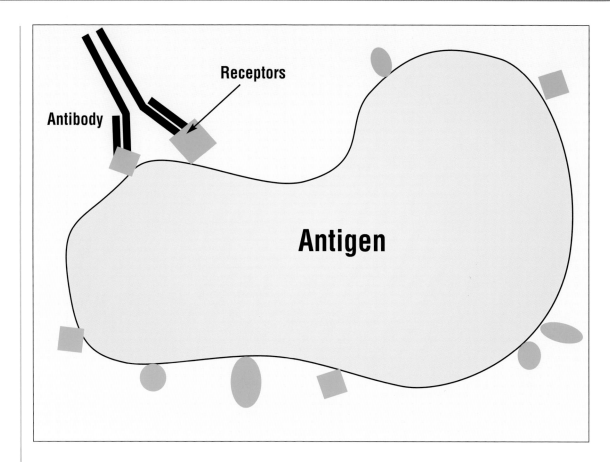

Lane TA. Leukocyte depletion of cellular blood components. *Curr Opin Hematol. 1994 Nov;1(6):443-51*

Anemia

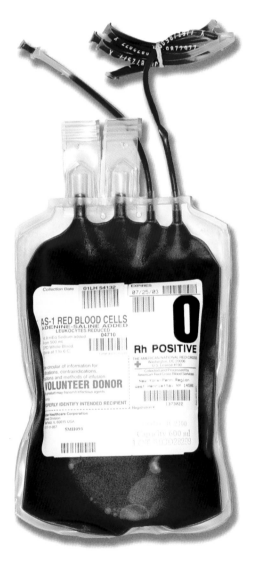

Patient:

Anemia is a condition caused by a lack of red blood cells. This condition may also exist when there are enough cells but they do not function correctly.

Clinical:

The World Health Organization defines anemia as a decrease in an individual's concentration of hemoglobin below that which is normal for that individual under ideal conditions. Generally, at sea level, a normal range for women is 12–16 grams of hemoglobin per deciliter of blood and 13–17 grams for men; anything below the range could be considered anemia. There are many different types of anemia. The most common being iron deficiency anemia that is caused by decreased levels of circulating and stored iron, resulting in red blood cells forming inadequately. This leads to less and often smaller than normal red blood cells that are lighter in color due to the lack of iron and hemoglobin. This condition is identified with a complete blood count and an iron profile test.

Freire WB. Strategies of the Pan American Health Organization/World Health Organization for the control of iron deficiency in Latin America. Nutr Rev. 1997 Jun;55(6):183-8.

It is the responsibility of the anesthesiologist to provide patients with a full evaluation before surgery, management of body systems during surgery, and care during their recovery from anesthesia.

It is very important that patients inform the surgeon of their wish to have bloodless surgery when scheduling the procedure to ensure adequate time for preparation. A "History and Physical" (a compilation of the patient's medical history and physical examination) and medical clearance for the procedure should be in place at least four weeks prior to the date of surgery. The anesthesiologist will work with the bloodless surgery coordinator and any involved physicians to ensure that medical conditions the patient may have are fully evaluated. For example, if a patient is anemic, the team would discuss options to strengthen the blood, increase iron, and raise hemoglobin levels. Each decision for therapy is tailor-made to the patient's needs, religious objections, and type of surgery.

The anesthesiologist will discuss with the patient several techniques that can be used in surgery to manage blood loss. Options include oxygen treatment, controlled hypotension, acute normovolemic hemodilution, cell salvage, volume expanders to replace lost blood, regional anesthesia, artificial blood substitutes (still experimental at this time, not routinely used), drugs to increase clotting effectiveness or to inhibit processes by which clots dissolve, patient positioning, and autologous blood.

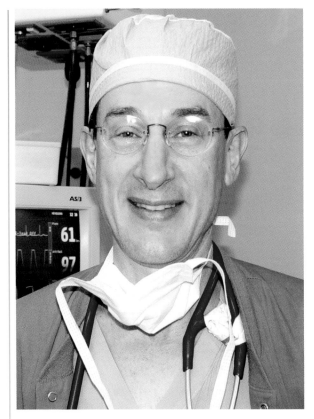

Shander A. Surgery without blood.
Crit Care Med. 2003 Dec;31(12 Suppl):S708-14.

Antibody

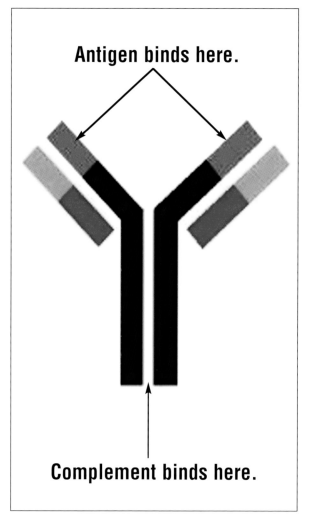

Antigen binds here.

Complement binds here.

Patient:

Substances produced in blood as a specific response to a particular antigen or allergen, such as a virus, germ, bacteria, or foreign protein. Antibodies can also exist naturally in the body, as in the case of immunoglobulins like IgA or IgE, which are considered to be "fractions" of blood.

Clinical:

A substance produced in blood that is capable of providing a specific immunity to a particular germ or virus. Proteins of the globulin class, most often gamma globulins, are produced by lymphocytes and plasma cells in response to antigenic stimulation. They may be specific, combining only with specific antigen molecules, or nonspecific, combining with a variety of antigens.

Tellier Z. Intravenous immunogloblins: myth and reality.
Isr Med Assoc J. 2005 Dec;7(12):762-7.7

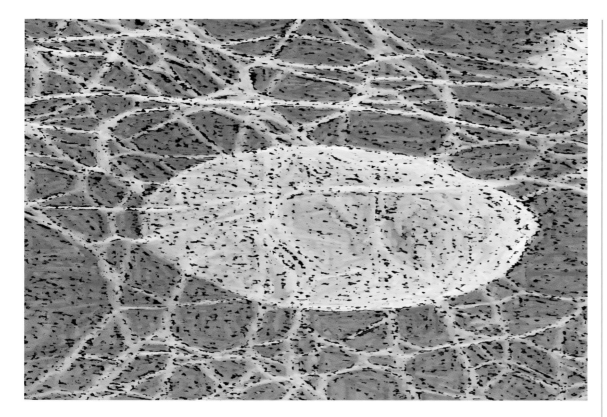

Patient:

A class of drugs that works to stop fibrinolysis, the breakdown of fibrin (a thready substance that holds clots together).

Clinical:

Stop fibrinolysis (the splitting up or dissolution of fibrin).

Serna DL, Thourani VH, Puskas JD. Antifibrinolytic agents in cardiac surgery: current controversies. Semin Thorac Cardiovasc Surg. 2005 Spring;17(1):52-8

Antigen

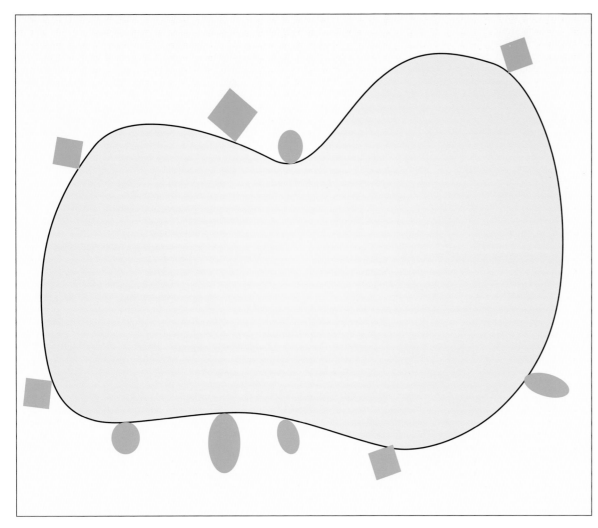

Patient:

Substances that produce an antibody response when they are introduced into the blood. Antigen-antibody response can make the body sensitive and/or resistant to various infections or toxic substances. Some common examples of antigens include pollen and poison ivy. Each blood group type has its own antigens, which is one reason why patients receiving a blood type that is not compatible with their own can be very dangerous.

Clinical:

An antigen is any substance that causes the formation of antibodies to it. The most common antigens are protein, but certain carbohydrate polysaccharides may act in a similar manner. Lipids may be combined with either. Each antigen has a certain chemical configuration that gives it antibody-provoking ability.

Westhoff CM, Reid ME. Review: the Kell, Duffy, and Kidd blood group systems. Immunohematol. 2004;20(1):37-49.

Yamamoto F. Review: ABO blood group system—ABH oligosaccharide antigens, anti-A and anti-B, A and B glycosyltransferases, and ABO genes. Immunohematol. 2004;20(1):3-22.

Autologous Blood

Patient:

The use of the patient's own blood to replace volume lost in surgery. There are two ways autologous blood can be used.

1. Provided the patient is not anemic, he or she donates blood several weeks before surgery at an interval of one to two times a week. The technician or nurse who withdraws the blood evaluates the patient's health before doing so, to ensure the safety of the procedure. Generally patients may donate more than once a week, with the last donation at least 72 hours before surgery, to allow the body's natural response to blood loss the time it needs to build up more red blood cells and restore the lost blood volume. Other conditions may preclude the patient's donating, such as a blood infection or the presence of certain viruses.

2. The second method is by acute normovolemic hemodilution (see pg. 60).

Clinical:

When patients donate their own blood prior to surgery for the use during or after the surgery. Preoperative autologous blood donation should be considered for elective surgical procedures during which significant blood loss may occur and for which blood would ordinarily be cross matched. The criteria for autologous donors are not as stringent as those for allogeneic donors. The Standards of the American Association of Blood Banks require that the donor-patients have a hemoglobin (Hb) of at least 11 g/dL and a hematocrit (HCT) of no less than 33% before each donation. There are no age or weight limits. Patients weighing 50 kg or more may donate 450±50 mL in addition to testing samples, whereas those weighing less than 50 kg can donate proportionately smaller volumes. Donations may be scheduled more than once a week, but the last should occur no less than 72 hours before surgery to allow time for restoration of intravascular volume and for the transport and testing of the donated blood. Donation is contraindicated when the patient has, or is being treated for, bacteremia or has a significant bacterial infection that can be associated with bacteremia. Blood center and transfusion service policies differ regarding collection and use of autologous blood with positive viral markers. However, it is common practice to preclude use of blood reactive for hepatitis B surface antigen and the human immunodeficiency virus because of concerns for the safety of both patients and personnel.

Goodnough LT. Autologous blood donation.
Anesthesiol Clin North America. 2005 Jun;23(2):263-70

Garcia-Erce JA, Munoz M, Bisbe E, Saez M, Solano VM, Beltran S, Ruiz A, Cuenca J, Vicente-Thomas J. Predeposit autologous donation in spinal surgery: a multicentre study. Eur Spine J. 2004 Oct;13 Suppl 1:S34-9. Epub 2004 Jul 6.

Autologous Cell Salvage

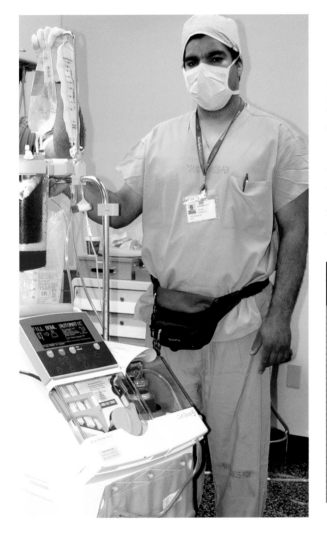

Patient:

A machine, commonly known as a cell saver, is used to recover red blood cells lost during surgery and return them to circulation in the patient's body. The first machine of this type was developed during the Vietnam War and used extensively in the field. This method may be acceptable for some of Jehovah's Witnesses.

Clinical:

The salvage of blood lost intraoperatively effectively minimizes the need for blood transfusion. This technique has had successful applications in various operative procedures, including cardiac surgery, spine surgery, liver transplantation, trauma procedures, and vascular surgery.

Autologous Cell Salvage—Jehovah's Witness Protocol:

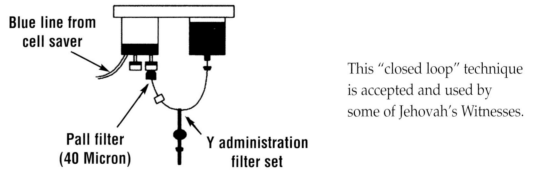

Blue line from cell saver

Pall filter (40 Micron)

Y administration filter set

This "closed loop" technique is accepted and used by some of Jehovah's Witnesses.

Waters JH. Indications and contraindications of cell salvage. Transfusion. 2004 Dec;44(12 Suppl):40S-4S.

Holt RL, Martin TD, Hess PJ, Beaver TM, Klodell CT. Jehovah's Witnesses requiring complex urgent cardiothoracic surgery. Ann Thorac Surg. 2004 Aug;78(2):695-7.

Reinfusion of a patient's own blood. In this picture, anesthesiologist Dr. Leon Basil transfuses blood that was collected and processed by a cell saver machine.

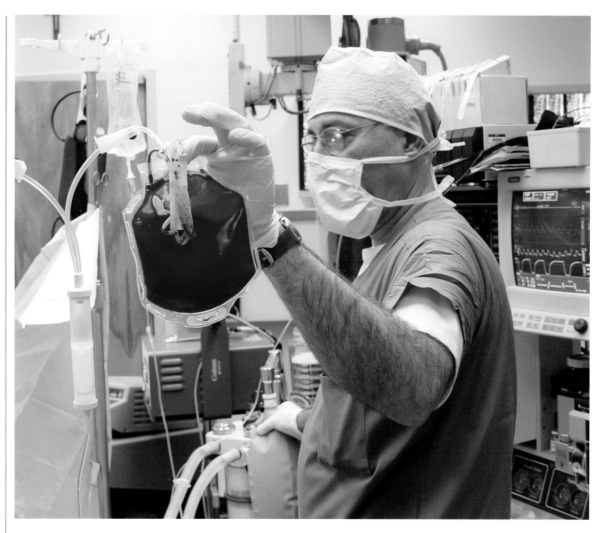

Chanda A, Smith DR, Nanda A. Autotransfusion by cell saver technique in surgery of lumbar and thoracic spinal fusion with instrumentation.
J Neurosurg. 2002 Apr;96(3 Suppl):298-303.

Waters JH. Red blood cell recovery and reinfusion.
Anesthesiol Clin North America. 2005 Jun;23(2):283-94

Blood Conservation

The science of minimizing blood loss through comprehensive patient evaluation, preoperative measures, and modern technology to both inhibit and salvage blood loss during surgery. Blood conservation techniques are necessary to perform "bloodless surgery" on patients who do not accept blood transfusions due to personal or religious reasons.

Some patients do not accept blood due to the risk of HIV, hepatitis, and other diseases. The number of patients with AIDS and various hepatitis viruses has been on the rise. These diseases and others could potentially be transferred during blood procedures. Due to these facts, some patients are avoiding the use of a blood transfusion. Most bloodless surgery programs offer the patient information and consultation on the safety of a blood transfusion during the surgery.

Patients who refuse blood for religious reasons, such as Jehovah's Witnesses, differ in acceptance of blood products and conservation techniques—particularly in the acceptance of cell salvage and the individual "fractions" or parts that comprise blood as a whole.

Holt RL, Martin TD, Hess PJ, Beaver TM, Klodell CT. Jehovah's Witnesses requiring complex urgent cardiothoracic surgery. Ann Thorac Surg. 2004 Aug;78(2):695-7.

Szpalski M, Gunzburg R, Sztern B. An overview of blood-sparing techniques used in spine surgery during the perioperative period. Eur Spine J. 2004 Oct;13 Suppl 1:S18-27. Epub 2004 Jun 15

Wade P. Treating Jehovah's Witnesses. Br J Perioper Nurs. 2004 Jun;14(6):254-7.

Sculco TP, Baldini A, Keating EM. Blood management in total joint arthroplasty. Instr Course Lect. 2005;54:51-66.

Blood Facts, Safety Data and International Issues

Today blood is safer than it has ever been, yet several safety concerns exist regarding blood transfusion.

1. **The effects of cold storage on blood and its ability to deliver oxygen to the tissues.** It can take up to 24 hours for red blood cells to regain their efficiency.

2. **Bacterial contamination of blood,** often due to inadequate preparation of the donor's arm—common with platelets.

3. **Human error.**

4. **The possibility for virus transmission** within the window of time between the discovery of a new virus and the development of an appropriate blood test. This problem has been addressed within blood banks all over the world. The risk is minimal.

One of the most recognized and well-documented side effects of a blood transfusion is immune suppression. This side effect can be averted by reducing the number of leukocytes (white blood cells) present in donated blood. This procedure is used in many hospitals abroad, but is not yet universal in the United States.

Medical institutions exhaust a considerable amount of funds preventing negative issues and supporting the continuous testing of blood. The cost of processing blood has increased dramatically. Presently, the cost of processing a unit of blood is approximately $500; this includes the costs of storage, testing, tubing, reagents, technicians, and other requirements.

Blood is often in short supply, and the trend is increasing. The American Red Cross announced that only 5% of the population donates blood, yet 76% expect it to be readily available. It is indicated that the type O– blood will not be available for elective surgeries. Blood drives and intensive efforts to educate the public are used to attract more blood donors. By the year 2030 the number of people needing blood transfusions is expected to double; thus the implementation of bloodless surgical procedures is imperative.

In the United States almost 13 million units of blood are used in one year; that equals *one half* of all the blood used elsewhere in the world. Regardless, the United States has to maintain its responsibility to conserve blood and help preserve its safe use for those who need it to survive.

Madjdpour C, Heindl V, Spahn DR.Risks, benefits, alternatives and indications of allogenic blood transfusions.

Minerva Anestesiol. 2006 May;72(5):283-98.
Zuck TF, Eyster ME. Blood safety decisions, 1982 to 1986: perceptions and misconceptions. Transfusion. 1996 Oct;36(10):928-31.

Sullivan P. Developing an administrative plan for transfusion medicine—a global perspective. Transfusion. 2005 Oct;45(4 Suppl):224S-40S.

Bloodless Surgery Coordinator

The person who assists the bloodless surgery team in organizing each patient's care plan and ensures that the patient's wishes are clearly stated and accurately documented. The coordinator will work with each patient to help identify potential complications with bloodless surgery (such as anemia) and assist the patient from the first visit to the surgeon's office to recovery at home. The coordinator will also assist with reimbursement issues when drugs such as erythropoietin alfa (EPO) are needed before surgery. A patient desiring bloodless surgery should contact the hospital to find out the availability of a blood conservation and/or bloodless surgery program. Bloodless programs have been adopted internationally because of the shortages and high cost of blood. Most patients who request bloodless surgery are Jehovah's Witnesses who refuse blood products for religious reasons. Courts have established statutes regarding the legal obligation. So hospitals and clinicians have to respect the wishes of every patient. In accordance, the patient first has to confirm his or her wishes regarding blood transfusion during the first visit to the surgeon.

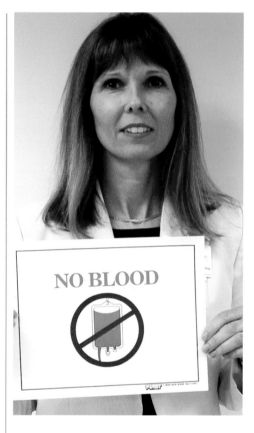

Rodriguez Moyado H. Bloodless medicine.
Rev Med Inst Mex Seguro Soc. 2005 May-Jun;43(3):229-35.

Bone marrow is an important part of the body that contains the precursor cells that generate new red and white blood cells in addition to platelets. The suppression of bone marrow function causes anemia; this suppression can be caused by chemotherapy or disease. The drug erythropoietin alfa (EPO) is used to stimulate the production of more red blood cells within bone marrow by mimicking the function of a naturally occurring substance in the body.

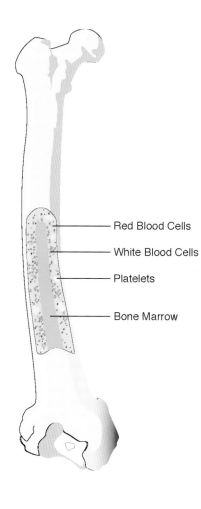

Red Blood Cells

White Blood Cells

Platelets

Bone Marrow

Beris P; Anemia Working Group. Erythropoietin and intravenous iron to save blood in surgerySchweiz Rundsch Med Prax. 2004 Nov 10;93(46):1905-10.

Colomina MJ, Bago J, Pellise F, Godet C, Villanueva C. Preoperative erythropoietin in spine surgery. Eur Spine J. 2004 Oct;13 Suppl 1:S40-9.

Coagulation

The process of blood clotting. A simple scab that forms on a knee, on the inside, is a complex bodily defense system. The defense system is designed to protect the vascular system, which is normally a closed loop. The body will use many "factors" to preserve the integrity of the vascular system: coagulation proteins, platelets, fibrin, fibrinogen, calcium, and thrombin. This knowledge is important because many of these components are derivatives of blood and may be considered part of Jehovah's Witnesses' conscience categories.

The process of blood clotting. It is a host defense procedure that maintains the integrity of the high-pressure closed circulatory system. After tissue is injured, alterations in the capillary bed and laceration of venules and arterioles lead to extravasation of blood into soft tissues or external bleeding. A platelet plug is formed through the processes of platelet adhesion and aggregation. To prevent excessive blood loss, the hemostatic system, which includes platelets, vascular endothelial cells, and plasma coagulation proteins, is invoked. Blood coagulation may be considered a mechanism for rapid replacement of an unstable platelet plug with a chemically stable fibrin clot.

Monroe DM, Hoffman M.
What does it take to make the perfect clot?
Arterioscler Thromb Vasc Biol. 2006 Jan;26(1):41-8. Epub 2005 Oct 27.

Hoffman MM, Monroe DM. Rethinking the coagulation cascade.
Curr Hematol Rep. 2005 Sep;4(5):391-6.

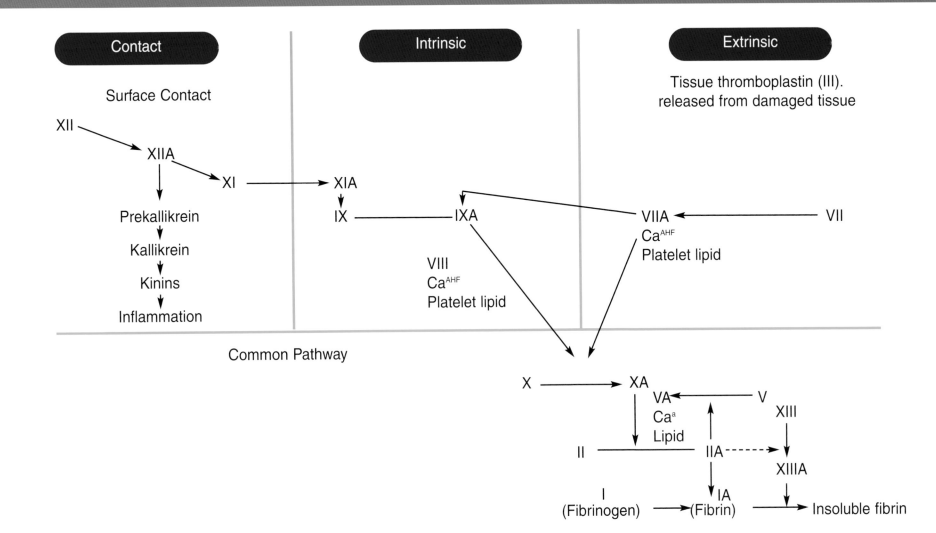

Colloids

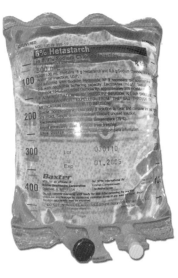

Patient:

Fluids that, like crystalloids, increase the volume within the vascular system by drawing fluid from patient's tissues into the bloodstream. Some colloids, such as albumin, are derived from blood whereas others like hetastarch, pentastarch, and dextran are nonblood volume expanders. Medical literature suggests that a combination of albumin and nonblood colloids can be effectively used.

Clinical:

Intravenous fluids used to maintain blood protein levels that stabilize fluid balances and circulation volume in the body. Some authors advocate the use of colloid solutions, such as albumin or hetastarch, because they may produce faster restoration of intravascular volume in traumatic shock. However, no convincing evidence demonstrates clear superiority of colloids over crystalloids in restoring volume depletion. Because colloids are more expensive, most physicians favor crystalloids unless serum albumin is low and requires repletion.

Boldt J, Suttner S. Plasma substitutes.
Minerva Anestesiol. 2005 Dec;71(12):741-58.

Bunn F, Alderson P, Hawkins V.
Colloid solutions for fluid resuscitation.
Cochrane Database Syst Rev. 2003;(1)

Cost of blood transfusion: An estimated unit of transfused blood cost $250 to process, $40 to type and screen, $42 to type and cross match, $75 in overhead (technicians, nurses, tubing, and office space, etc.), and $100 for pathogen reduction (if implemented). The total is approximately $500 per unit.

The total cost for blood transfusion in the United States has been estimated at between **$1 and $2 billion** per year.

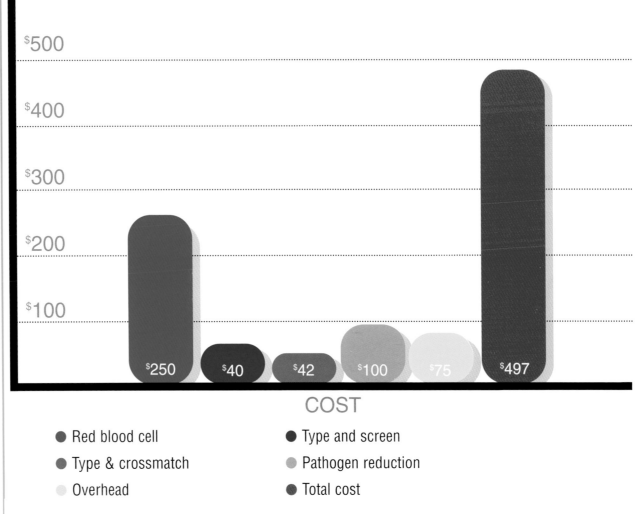

	COST

- ● Red blood cell
- ● Type & crossmatch
- ● Overhead
- ● Type and screen
- ● Pathogen reduction
- ● Total cost

Liberman A, Rotarius T. A new cost allocation method for hospital-based clinical laboratories and transfusion services: implications for transfusion medicine. Transfusion. 2005 Oct;45(10):1684-8.

Spence RK. Blood management in orthopaedic surgery. Instr Course Lect. 2005;54:43-9

Cryoprecipitates

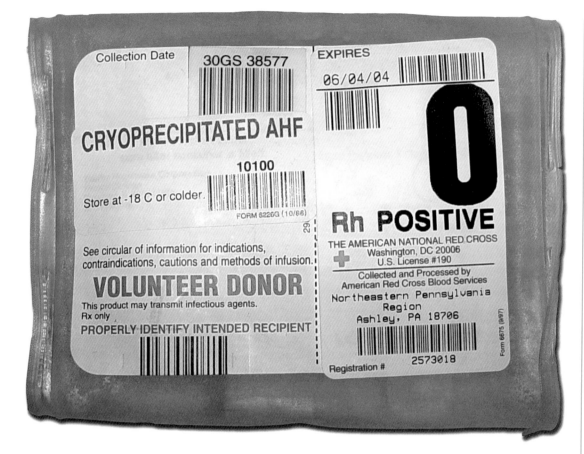

Collection Date 30GS 38577

EXPIRES 06/04/04

CRYOPRECIPITATED AHF

10100

Store at -18 C or colder.

FORM 6226G (10/86)

See circular of information for indications, contraindications, cautions and methods of infusion.

VOLUNTEER DONOR

This product may transmit infectious agents.
Rx only

PROPERLY IDENTIFY INTENDED RECIPIENT

0

Rh POSITIVE

THE AMERICAN NATIONAL RED CROSS
Washington, DC 20006
U.S. License #190

Collected and Processed by
American Red Cross Blood Services
Northeastern Pennsylvania
Region
Ashley, PA 18706

Form 6675 (3/97)

Registration # 2573018

Patient:

The substances that form when frozen blood plasma is thawed. During the thawing procedure, the frozen plasma is placed in a centrifuge and is separated into its various parts; the resulting derivatives, or "precipitates," contain an important clotting Factor VIII (antihemophilic), some Factor XIII, fibrinogen, and von Willebrand's factor. Cryoprecipitates are a fraction of blood that may be acceptable for use by Jehovah's Witnesses.

Clinical:

A small portion of plasma that contains specific clotting factors. If bleeding is caused by a deficiency in clotting factors, cryoprecipitates are generally infused to correct the bleeding problem. This product may be recommended for treatment of deficiencies of Factor VIII, Factor XIII, and fibrinogen.

Farrugia A, Robert P. Plasma protein therapies: current and future perspectives.
Best Pract Res Clin Haematol. 2006;19(1):243-58

Patient:

Fluids that, like colloids, increase the volume within the vascular system by drawing fluid from patient's tissues into the bloodstream. However, unlike colloids, crystalloids can pass through semi-permeable membranes such as blood vessels. The anesthesiologist determines the best fluid combinations for a patient based on how much fluid the heart can tolerate, how much blood is lost, what kind of surgery is performed, and whether the patient accepts minor fractions of blood.

Clinical:

Fluids that contain water and electrolytes. They are grouped as balanced, hypertonic, and hypotonic salt solutions. Crystalloid solutions are used to maintain water and electrolytes, and expand intravascular fluid. Administered crystalloid is distributed in a 1:4 ratio. It is the same as extracellular fluid, which is composed of about 3 liters of intravascularly (plasma) and about 12 liters of extravascular fluid. The replacement requirement is 3- or 4-fold the volume of blood lost.

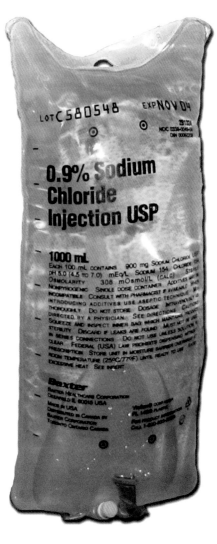

Moore EE, Johnson JL, Cheng AM, Masuno T, Banerjee A. Insights from studies of blood substitutes in trauma. Shock. 2005 Sep;24(3):197-205.

Gould SA, Sehgal LR, Sehgal HL, Moss GS. Hypovolemic shock. Crit Care Clin. 1993 Apr;9(2):239-59.

Dextran

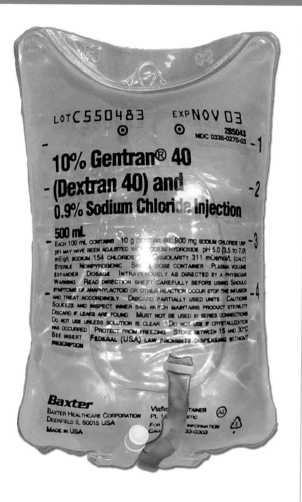

Patient:

A non-blood volume expander. (See pg. 80 for information on colloids.) Dextran is typically used in cases with moderate or severe blood loss to maintain the pressure in arteries and veins.

Clinical:

An intravenous fluid used to increase plasma volume, venous return, and cardiac output. Dextran is available as either Dextran 40 or Dextran 70; the numbers 40 and 70 refer to the average molecular weight in the solution. The Dextran solutions are water-soluble glucose polymers synthesized by certain bacteria from sucrose. Dextran 40 and 70 are ultimately degraded enzymatically to glucose. A colloid solution of 6% Dextran 70 is administered for the same indications as 5% albumin.

Moore FA, McKinley BA, Moore EE.
The next generation in shock resuscitation.
Lancet. 2004 Jun 12;363(9425):1988-96.

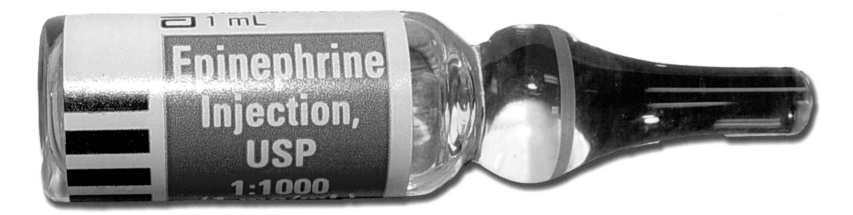

Patient:

A chemical commonly used to constrict blood vessels in the vicinity of a surgical incision. The constriction of the blood vessels results in less bleeding during the skin incision of the operation.

Clinical:

A potent activator of adrenergic receptors. The activation of alpha receptors produces vasoconstriction in the epinephrine is available in local anesthetics such as lidocaine with epinephrine or as adrenalin chloride solution. It is inexpensive and readily available.

Kopacz DJ, Helman JD, Nussbaum CE, Hsiang JN, Nora PC, Allen HW. A comparison of epidural levobupivacaine 0.5% with or without epinephrine for lumbar spine surgery. Anesth Analg. 2001 Sep;93(3):755-60.

Erythropoietin

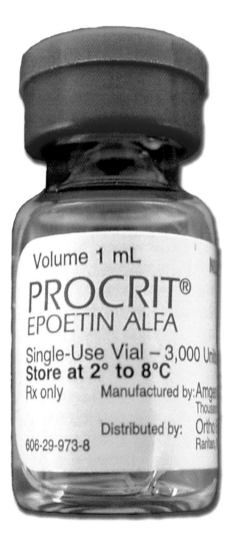

Volume 1 mL

PROCRIT®
EPOETIN ALFA

Single-Use Vial – 3,000 U
Store at 2° to 8°C
Rx only   Manufactured by:Amge
                            Thous
           Distributed by: Ortho
606-29-973-8   Rarita

Patient:

A substance used to increase the amount of red blood cells produced by the body's bone marrow. With the availability of epoetin alfa, there has been a decrease in the need for blood and blood donation.

Clinical:

A glycoprotein that acts on the bone marrow to selectively increase erythropoiesis. It is produced predominantly when the body responds to low oxygen levels. Erythropointin is formed in the kidney, but extrarenal production sites such as the liver has been identified. Epoetin alfa, the name selected for the recombinant human erythropoietin, is now commercially available. It is commonly used to treat anemia associated with renal insufficiency and has been successfully used for patients refusing blood transfusion for religious reasons. Few adverse effects can include hypertension, seizures, and thrombotic events. Increased mortality and or tumor progression has been reported in patients with active malignant disease.

*Shapiro GS, Boachie-Adjei O, Dhawlikar SH, Maier LS.
The use of Epoetin alfa in complex spine deformity surgery.
Spine. 2002 Sep 15;27(18):2067-71.*

Patient:

Substances that serve as tissue adhesive, or "glue." They are designed to mimic the final steps of blood coagulation and consequently assist in the process of wound healing, and sometimes in the sealing of dural repairs.

Clinical:

Derived from plasma products and contain fibrinogen, thrombin, an antifibrinolytic agent "aprotinin." and calcium chloride. Some fibrin sealants also contain Factor XIII.

Tredwell SJ, Sawatzky B. The use of fibrin sealant to reduce blood loss during Cotrel-Dubousset instrumentation for idiopathic scoliosis. Spine. 1990 Sep;15(9):913-5.

Lee MG, Jones D. Applications of fibrin sealant in surgery. Surg Innov. 2005 Sep;12(3):203-13.

Fibrinogen

Patient:

A critical component in the clotting of blood (also known as Factor I).

Clinical:

The soluble fibrinogen molecule is converted into soluble fibrin during the process of blood coagulation. The polymerized fibrin serves as a template for the localized assembly and activation of the fibrinolytic system, which modulates fibrin deposition and clot dissolution.

Mayer PJ, Gehlsen JA. Coagulopathies associated with major spinal surgery.
Clin Orthop Relat Res. 1989 Aug;(245):83-8

Members of the vitamin B complex that are components of the red blood cell production process. Folate occurs naturally in food; folic acid is the synthetic form and it is found in supplements and fortified foods. Adults and children need folate to maintain a normal level of red blood cells and to prevent anemia. Folate can be found in leafy green vegetables, liver, lentils, black-eyed peas, beans, citrus, strawberries and certain tropical fruits.

Supplementation of folic acid is recommended in cases of anemia. Do not take it if you have pernicious anemia or if you are on anticoagulation medication.

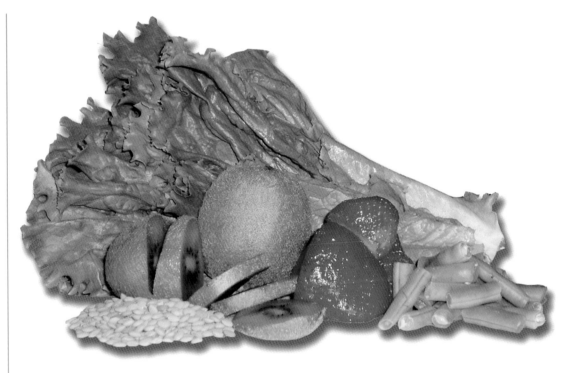

Proposito D, Gramolini R, Corazza V, Mancini B, Gallina S, Montemurro L, Veltri S, Carboni M. Objectives of a bloodless surgery program. A comparative study (major surgery vs. minor-medium surgery) in 51 Jehova's Witnesses patients Ann Ital Chir. 2002 Mar-Apr;73(2):197-209

Gelatin

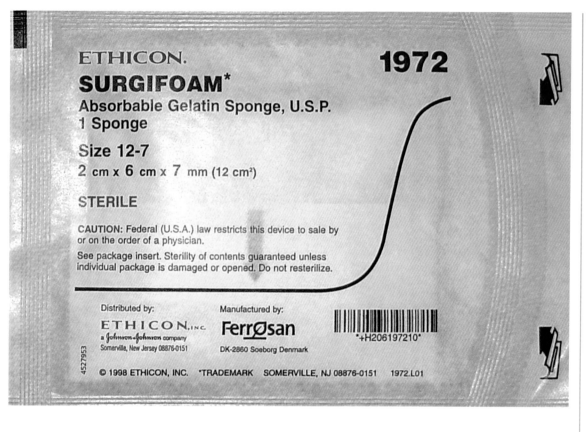

ETHICON.

SURGIFOAM*

Absorbable Gelatin Sponge, U.S.P.
1 Sponge

Size 12-7

2 cm x 6 cm x 7 mm (12 cm²)

STERILE

CAUTION: Federal (U.S.A.) law restricts this device to sale by
or on the order of a physician.

See package insert. Sterility of contents guaranteed unless
individual package is damaged or opened. Do not resterilize.

1972

Distributed by:

ETHICON,INC.
a Johnson-Johnson company
Somerville, New Jersey 08876-0151

Manufactured by:

FerrØsan

DK-2860 Soeborg Denmark

H206197210

4527953

© 1998 ETHICON, INC.   *TRADEMARK   SOMERVILLE, NJ 08876-0151   1972.L01

Gelatin is used during surgery to slow blood secretion and allow blood clots to form. Gelatin can be applied to a wound bed in the form of a powder or a sponge. Spinal surgeons use this material to gently pack and stop bleeding around the dura and by the nerve roots.

Aziz O, Athanasiou T, Darzi A. Haemostasis using a ready-to-use collagen sponge coated with activated thrombin and fibrinogen. Surg Technol Int. 2005;14:35-40.

Hemoglobin is the critical component that enables red blood cells to carry oxygen from the lungs throughout the entire body.

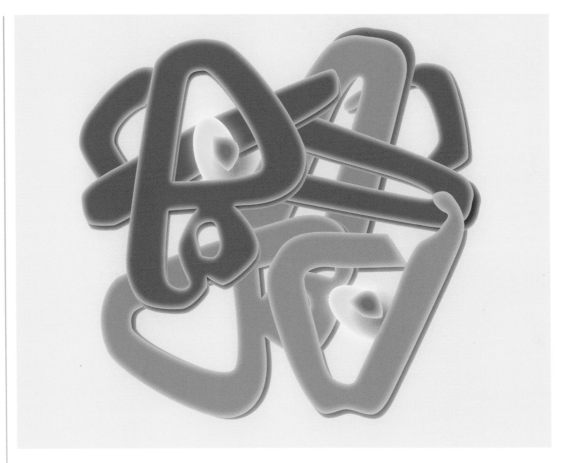

Madjdpour C, Heindl V, Spahn DR. Risks, benefits, alternatives and indications of allogenic blood transfusions. Minerva Anestesiol. 2006 May;72(5):283-98.

Hetastarch

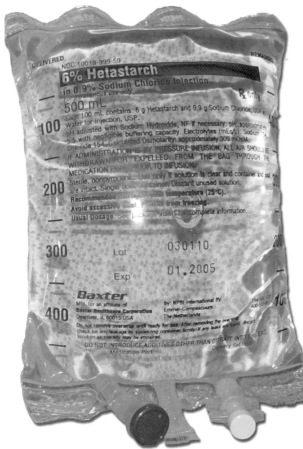

Patient:

A nonblood volume expander. (see colloids on pg. 80). Hetastarch may be used in cases with moderate or severe blood loss, to maintain the pressure in arteries and veins.

Fenger-Eriksen C, Hartig Rasmussen C, Kappel Jensen T, Anker-Moller E, Heslop J, Frokiaer J, Tonnesen E. Renal effects of hypotensive anaesthesia in combination with acute normovolaemic haemodilution with hydroxyethyl starch 130/0.4 or isotonic saline. Acta Anaesthesiol Scand. 2005 Aug;49(7):969-74.

Simon J, Jung F, Holbach T, Castor G, Jaksche H, Kiesewetter H. Intra- and postoperative effect of various plasma substitutes on blood rheology and conjunctival oxygen partial pressure in micro-surgical intervertebral disk operations. Infusionstherapie. 1989 Feb;16(1):30-8.

Clinical:

An intravenous fluid used as a volume expander. Hydroxyethyl starch (hetastarch) is a synthetic colloid solution in which the molecular weight of at least 80% of the polymers ranges from 10,000 to 2,000,000. It is available in the United States as a 6% solution in 0.9% sodium chloride (Hespan). It produces dilutional effects similar to other volume expanders. Hetastarch reduces Factor VIII C levels by 50% in a dose of 1 L with prolongation of the partial thromboplastin time. It can interfere with clot formation by direct movement of hetastarch molecules into the fibrin clot. There are a number of different molecular weight hetastarch products around the world; however, only products with a high molecular weight (450,000–800,000) are available in the United States.

Blood that is taken from one person and given to another (also referred to as allogenic or banked blood). Donated blood is coded using the A-B-O and Rh grouping systems, which determine the compatibility of the donor and recipient.

Some members of the team to the right may have type AB+; they are universal recipients and can safely receive any blood type. Others may have type O–; they are universal donors whose blood can safely be transfused to a recipient with a different blood type.

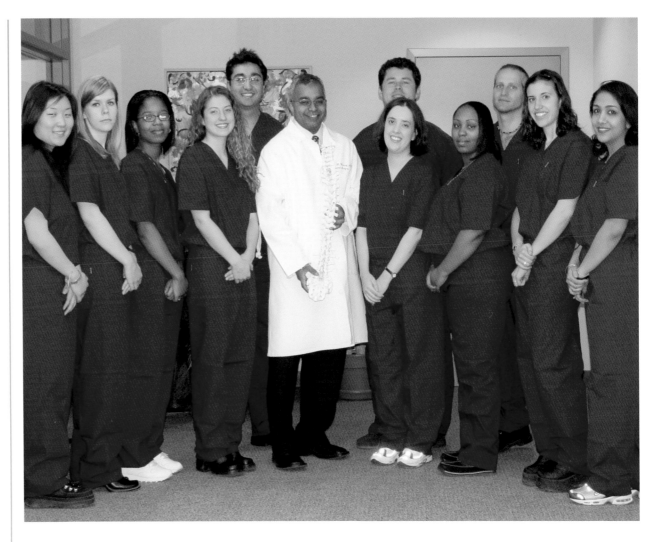

Szpalski M, Gunzburg R, Sztern B. An overview of blood-sparing techniques used in spine surgery during the perioperative period. Eur Spine J. 2004 Oct;13 Suppl 1:S18-27. Epub 2004 Jun 15.

Iron Supplementation

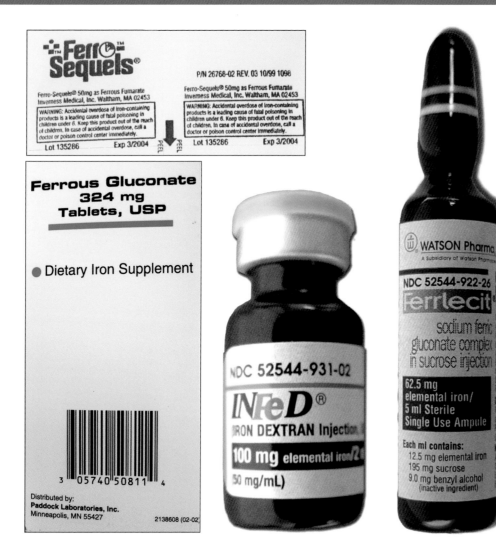

An oral medication containing either ferrous gluconate or ferrous sulfate. Iron supplementation is an inexpensive and generally well tolerated treatment often used for iron-deficiency anemia. Possible side effects of iron supplementation include constipation, diarrhea, and a false-positive result on occult fecal blood test.

Proposito D, Gramolini R, Corazza V, Mancini B, Gallina S, Montemurro L, Veltri S, Carboni M. Objectives of a bloodless surgery program. A comparative study (major surgery vs. minor-medium surgery) in 51 Jehovah's Witnesses patients Ann Ital Chir. 2002 Mar-Apr;73(2):197-209

Excellent Food Sources

- Beef
- Oysters
- Calf/beef liver
- Sardines
- Pork
- Clams
- Turkey
- Salmon
- Veal
- Tuna
- Chicken
- Scallops
- Chicken liver
- Mackarel
- Lamb

Vegetarian Options

- Spinach
- Branflakes
- Almonds
- Muesli
- Baked Beans

Good Food Sources

- Iron-fortified cereals
- Brown rice
- Peanut Butter
- Eggs

Greens

- Dandelion
- Turnips
- Collard
- Spinach
- Mustard
- Beets
- Swiss Chard

Beans

- Lima
- Peas
- Black beans
- Molasses
- Lentils
- Soybeans

Dried Fruits

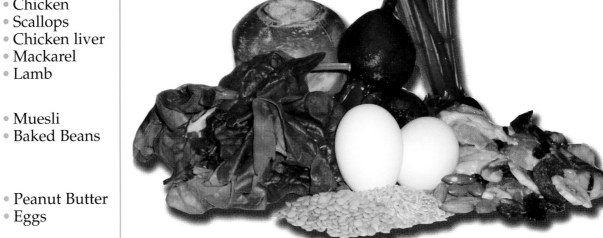

Lopez MA, Martos FC. Iron availability: An updated review. Int J Food Sci Nutr. 2004 Dec;55(8):597-606.

Leukocytes

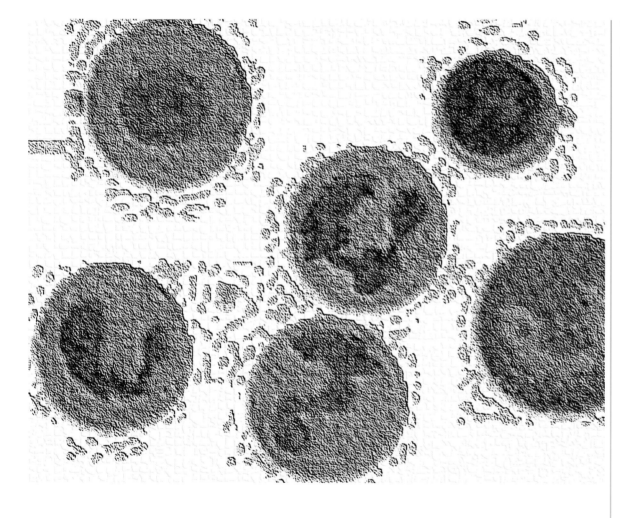

White blood cells are made by the bone marrow. These cells fight infection.

Vamvakas EC, Blajchman MA. Universal WBC reduction: the case for and against. Transfusion. 2001 May;41(5):691-712.

Patient:

Applied directly to a wound and held in place to stop bleeding during surgery.

Clinical:

Prepared by mechanically breaking down bovine collagen into fibrils. Available in both fibrous (granular) and web forms, fibrous collagen is applied directly to the wound and held in place. The highly effective collagen produces aggregate platelets on their surface. Avitene is a fibrous form of collagen, which is offered by Alcon Laboratories (Fort Worth, Texas).

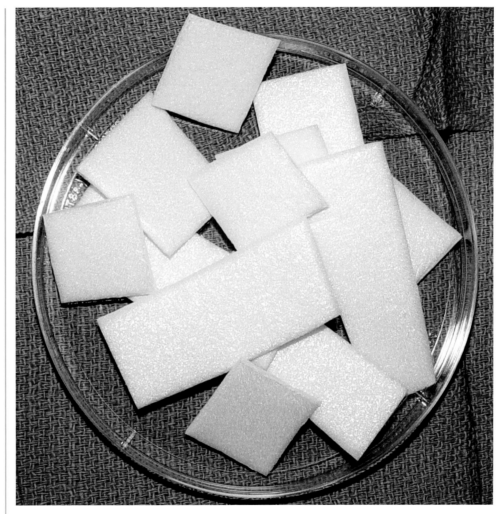

Larson PO. Topical hemostatic agents for dermatologic surgery.
J Dermatol Surg Oncol. 1988 Jun;14(6):623-32.

Normal Saline

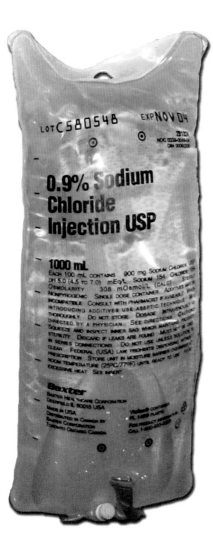

LOT C580548 EXP NOV 04

0.9% Sodium
Chloride
Injection USP

1000 mL

Normal saline solution is one of the most widely used intravenous solutions. This solution is considered to be isotonic and isosomotic.

Spence RK, Parce P. Perioperative assessment of the elective orthopedic surgery patient. Anesthesiol Clin North America. 2005 Jun;23(2):295-303

Patient:

Absorbable fiber that inhibits blood flow and assists with blood clotting when applied to a wound.

Clinical:

An absorbable fiber prepared from cellulose. Woven strips of cellulose are cut and held with firm pressure on the wound bed, causing local vasoconstriction and providing a meshwork for coagulation. Surgicel is offered by Johnson and Johnson (Arlington, Texas)

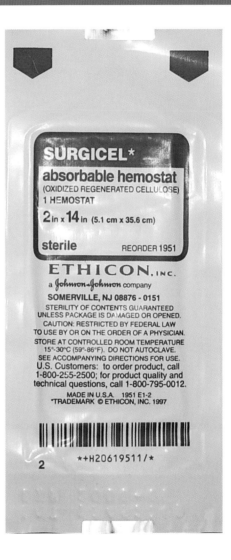

Larson PO. Topical hemostatic agents for dermatologic surgery. J Dermatol Surg Oncol. 1988 Jun;14(6):623-32.

Pentastarch

Patient:

A nonblood volume expander (see Colloids on pg. 80). Pentastarch may be used in cases with moderate or severe blood loss, to maintain the fluid pressure in arteries and veins.

Clinical:

The colloidal properties of pentastarch are used as a plasma volume expander. Intravenous infusion of pentastarch results in the expansion of the plasma volume in excess of the volume infused. This expansion persists for approximately 18 to 24 hours and is expected to improve the hemodynamic status for 12 to 18 hours.

Pentastarch molecules below 50,000 molecular weight are rapidly eliminated by renal excretion. A single dose of approximately 500 mL results in the elimination, by urine, of approximately 70% of the dose within 24 hours and approximately 80% of the dose within one week. The remaining percentage of the administered dose is presumed to be eliminated at a slower rate. This process is variable and generally results in an intravascular pentastarch concentration below the level of detection by one week.

Indications and Clinical Uses:

Pentastarch is used when plasma volume expansion is desired as an adjunct in the management of shock due to hemorrhage, surgery, sepsis, burns or other trauma. It is not a substitute for red blood cells or coagulation factors in plasma.

Contraindications:

Patients with hypersensitivity to hydroxyethyl starch, with bleeding disorders, or with congestive heart failure where volume overload is a potential problem. Pentastarch should not be used if renal disease is present.

Kozek-Langenecker SA. Effects of hydroxyethyl starch solutions on hemostasis. Anesthesiology. 2005 Sep;103(3):654-60.

Jungheinrich C, Neff TA. Pharmacokinetics of hydroxyethyl starch. Clin Pharmacokinet. 2005;44(7):681-99.

Patient:

Perfluorochemicals (PFCs) have the potential ability to perform the red blood cell's function of transporting oxygen and carbon dioxide throughout the body. Presently, these products are still in development.

Clinical:

Perfluorochemicals have the ability to carry oxygen and carbon dioxide; the use of PFCs is currently being tested. Perfluorocarbons dissolve more oxygen than any other inert liquid. Better results can be obtained using phospho-lipid-stabilized emulsions. Lower inspired oxygen levels and higher con-centrations of perfluorochemicals are possible. Further developments of blood substitutes are being performed. As a result Oxygent and Liquivent are being produced and investigated by Alliance.

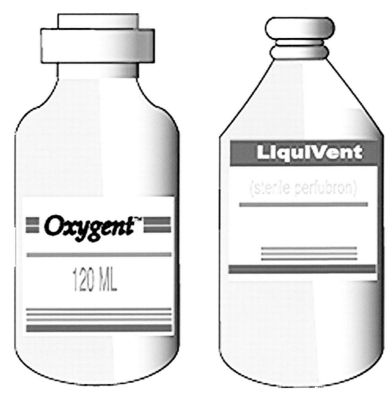

101. Perfluorochemicals
Habler O, Pape A, Meier J, Zwissler B. Artificial oxygen carriers as an alternative to red blood cell transfusion. Anaesthesist. 2005 Aug;54(8):741-54.

Lowe KC. Engineering blood: synthetic substitutes from fluorinated compounds. Tissue Eng. 2003 Jun;9(3):389-99.

Chang TM. Future generations of red blood cell substitutes. J Intern Med. 2003 May;253(5):527-35.

Gaudard A, Varlet-Marie E, Bressolle F, Audran M. Drugs for increasing oxygen and their potential use in doping: a review. Sports Med. 2003;33(3):187-212.

Klein HG.Blood substitutes: how close to a solution? Oncology (Williston Park). 2002 Sep;16(9 Suppl 10):147-51.

Plasma (FFP)

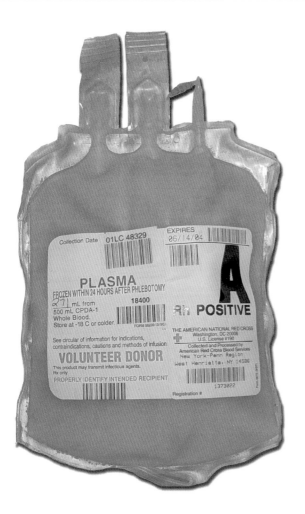

The liquid portion of blood. When blood is obtained from a donor, the plasma is extracted from the blood and then frozen. Plasma contains proteins (Factors V and VIII) that gradually decline over the duration of the blood's storage.

MacLennan S, Barbara JA. Risks and side effects of therapy with plasma and plasma fractions. Best Pract Res Clin Haematol. 2006;19(1):169-89.

McLeod BC. Therapeutic apheresis: use of human serum albumin, fresh frozen plasma and cryosupernatant plasma in therapeutic plasma exchange. Best Pract Res Clin Haematol. 2006;19(1):157-67.

Patient:

The portion of blood that is essential in the formation of blood clots. Aspirin irreversibly damages platelets, which are gradually replaced by the body over the course of approximately ten days.

Clinical:

Small structures in blood that assist blood clotting. Normal clotting includes platelet hemostatic plug formation and fibrin production phases. The fibrin production phase occurs by either intrinsic or extrinsic pathways. Acquired platelet abnormalities include problems of decreased production and function, in addition to increased destruction.

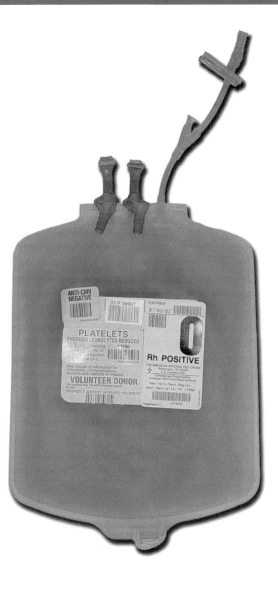

Pietrzak WS, Eppley BL. Platelet rich plasma: biology and new technology.
J Craniofac Surg. 2005 Nov;16(6):1043-54.

Red Blood Cells

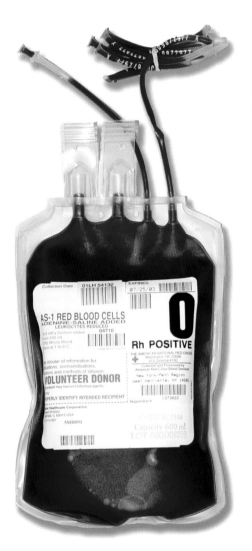

Red blood cells are also called erythrocytes. They serve two important functions:

1. The transport of oxygen from the lungs to cells throughout the body. (Oxygen is used to obtain energy from food.)

2. The transport of carbon dioxide from the cells to the lungs. (Carbon dioxide is released as a waste product of cell processes.)

Hogman CF, Meryman HT. Red blood cells intended for transfusion: quality criteria revisited. Transfusion. 2006 Jan;46(1):137-42.

A nonblood volume expander used in cases of acute blood loss (see Crystalloids page 83). Ringer's lactated solution is considered a more physiologic replacement than normal saline solution.

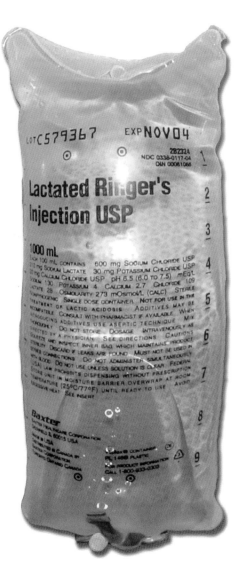

Glover JL, Broadie TA.Intraoperative autotransfusion.
Prog Clin Biol Res. 1982;108:151-70.

Thrombin

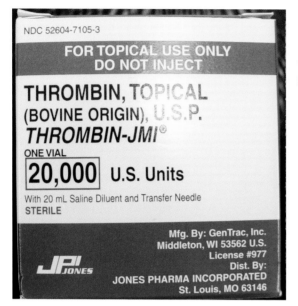

NDC 52604-7105-3

**FOR TOPICAL USE ONLY
DO NOT INJECT**

THROMBIN, TOPICAL
(BOVINE ORIGIN), U.S.P.
THROMBIN-JMI®

ONE VIAL
20,000 U.S. Units

With 20 mL Saline Diluent and Transfer Needle
STERILE

Mfg. By: GenTrac, Inc.
Middleton, WI 53562 U.S.
License #977
Dist. By:
JONES PHARMA INCORPORATED
St. Louis, MO 63146

Patient:

A potent clotting agent that is used to stop bleeding during surgery.

Clinical:

A freeze-dried powder that can be applied directly to a wound bed or mixed with isotonic saline to be administered by sponge or spray. The wound bed should be sponged free of excess blood before thrombin is applied. Thrombin does not injure tissue or produce residue on the tissue bed. Once the solution is prepared, it must be used within 6 hours. Thrombin is very expensive and the high cost prohibits its routine use in office procedures.

Larson PO. Topical hemostatic agents for dermatologic surgery.
J Dermatol Surg Oncol. 1988 Jun;14(6):623-32.

This vitamin promotes cell repair and growth, and it maintains the integrity of the nervous system. It is difficult to consume low amounts of vitamin B12; therefore, a deficiency may not be a result of poor diet but rather the body's difficulty in absorbing the vitamin during digestion. The body's inability to absorb sufficient amounts of vitamin B12 could be due to low levels of hydrochloric acid; consequently patients who suffer from gastritis are prone to deficiency. Poor absorption can also be caused by the absence of a specific glycoprotein that attaches to vitamin B12 and aids in digestion. This condition is known as pernicious anemia. Patients who have difficulty absorbing vitamin B12 must be intra-muscularly injected with the vitamin, thus bypassing the digestive system.

Do not take vitamin B12 if you have atrophy of the optic nerve.

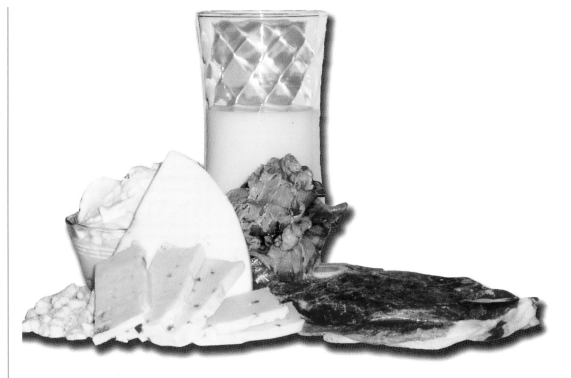

Ho C, Kauwell GP, Bailey LB Practitioners' guide to meeting the vitamin B-12 recommended dietary allowance for people aged 51 years and older.
J Am Diet Assoc. 1999 Jun;99(6):725-7.

Vitamin C Food Sources

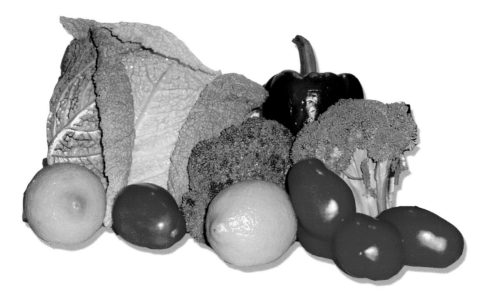

Recommendations for supplementation should be made by a physician.

- Currants
- Kale
- Cabbage
- Hot Peppers
- Sweet Peppers

- Tomato
- Broccoli
- Green Peppers
- Lemons
- Tangerines

- Guava
- Strawberries
- Papaya

An important function of vitamin C is the formation and maintenance of collagen. Collagen is the basis of connective tissue found in skin, ligaments, cartilage, vertebral discs, joint linings, capillary walls, bones, and teeth. It is needed to give support and shape to the body, heal wounds, and maintain healthy blood vessels.

Vitamin C is an antioxidant vitamin. It helps prevent the creation of free radicals that generate cellular injury and disease.

Vitamin C has been shown, through research, to stimulate the immune system. Ascorbic acid (found in vitamin C) may activate neutrophils, the most prevalent white blood cells that are the front-line defense of the immune system. Functioning as an antioxidant, vitamin C helps in the prevention and treatment of infections and other diseases.

McDermott JH. Antioxidant nutrients: current dietary recommendations and research update. J Am Pharm Assoc (Wash). 2000 Nov-Dec;40(6):785-99.

Selected References

HERNIATED NUCLEUS PULPOSUS

Boden SD, Davis DO, Dina TS, Patronas NJ, Wiesel SW.: Abnormal magnetic-resonance scans of the lumbar spine in asymptomatic subjects. A prospective investigation.
J Bone Joint Surg Am. 1990 Mar;72(3):403-8.

Kawakami M, Tamaki T, Hayashi N, Hashizume H, Nishi H.: Possible mechanism of painful radiculopathy in lumbar disc herniation.
Clin Orthop Relat Res. 1998 Jun;(351):241-51.

Konttinen YT, Kemppinen P, Li TF, Waris E, Pihlajamaki H, Sorsa T, Takagi M, Santavirta S, Schultz GS, Humphreys-Beher MG.:Transforming and epidermal growth factors in degenerated intervertebral discs.
J Bone Joint Surg Br. 1999 Nov;81(6):1058-63.

Burke JG, Watson RW, McCormack D, Dowling FE, Walsh MG, Fitzpatrick JM.Intervertebral discs which cause low back pain secrete high levels of proinflammatory mediators.
J Bone Joint Surg Br. 2002 Mar;84(2):196-201.

Kawakami M, Matsumoto T, Tamaki T.: Roles of thromboxane A2 and leukotriene B4 in radicular pain induced by herniated nucleus pulposus.
J Orthop Res. 2001 May;19(3):472-7.

Yabuki S.Basic and update knowledge of intervertebral disc herniation: review.
Fukushima J Med Sci. 1999 Dec;45(2):63-75.

Takahashi N, Yabuki S, Aoki Y, Kikuchi S.: Pathomechanisms of nerve root injury caused by disc herniation: an experimental study of mechanical compression and chemical irritation.
Spine. 2003 Mar 1;28(5):435-41.

Pope MH, Magnusson M, Wilder DG.:Kappa Delta Award. Low back pain and whole body vibration.
Clin Orthop Relat Res. 1998 Sep;(354):241-8.

Pecha MD.: Herniated nucleus pulposus as a result of emesis in a 20-yr-old man.
Am J Phys Med Rehabil. 2004 Apr;83(4):327-30.

Schneider M, Santolin S, Farrell P.:False negative magnetic resonance imaging results: a report of 2 cases.
J Manipulative Physiol Ther. 2005 May;28(4):278-84.

Marion PJ, Kahanovitz N.: Lumbar-sacral radiculopathy secondary to intraspinal synovial cyst.
Arch Phys Med Rehabil. 1995 Nov;76(11):1011-3.

Sculco AD, Paup DC, Fernhall B, Sculco MJ.:Effects of aerobic exercise on low back pain patients in treatment.
Spine J. 2001 Mar-Apr;1(2):95-101.

Saal JS, Saal JA, Yurth EF.: Nonoperative management of herniated cervical intervertebral disc with radiculopathy.
Spine. 1996 Aug 15;21(16):1877-83.

Vad VB, Bhat AL, Lutz GE, Cammisa F.:Transforaminal epidural steroid injections in lumbosacral radiculopathy: a prospective randomized study.
Spine. 2002 Jan 1;27(1):11-6.

Buttermann GR.: Treatment of lumbar disc herniation: epidural steroid injection compared with discectomy. A prospective, randomized study.
J Bone Joint Surg Am. 2004 Apr;86-A(4):670-9.

Eriksen K.: Management of cervical disc herniation with upper cervical chiropractic care.
J Manipulative Physiol Ther. 1998 Jan;21(1):51-6.

Benoist M.: The natural history of lumbar disc herniation and radiculopathy.
Joint Bone Spine. 2002 Mar;69(2):155-60.

Chiu JC, Clifford TJ, Greenspan M, Richley RC, Lohman G, Sison RB.: Percutaneous microdecompressive endoscopic cervical discectomy with laser thermodiskoplasty.
Mt Sinai J Med. 2000 Sep;67(4):278-82.

Regan JJ, Mack MJ, Picetti GD 3rd.: A technical report on video-assisted thoracoscopy in thoracic spinal surgery. Preliminary description.
Spine. 1995 Apr 1;20(7):831-7.

Ikard RW, McCord DH.: Thoracoscopic exposure of intervertebral discs.
Ann Thorac Surg. 1996 Apr;61(4):1267-8.

Choy DS.: Percutaneous laser disc decompression (PLDD): twelve years' experience with 752 procedures in 518 patients.
J Clin Laser Med Surg. 1998 Dec;16(6):325-31.

Iwatsuki K, Yoshimine T, Sasaki M, Yasuda K, Akiyama C, Nakahira R. The effect of laser irradiation for nucleus pulposus: an experimental study.
Neurol Res. 2005 Apr;27(3):319-23.

Mathews HH, Long BH.: Minimally invasive techniques for the treatment of intervertebral disk herniation.
J Am Acad Orthop Surg. 2002 Mar-Apr;10(2):80-5.

Errico TJ, Fardon DF, Lowell TD.: Open discectomy as treatment for herniated nucleus pulposus of the lumbar spine.
Spine. 1995 Aug 15;20(16):1829-33.

Watkins RG 4th, Williams LA, Watkins RG 3rd.: Microscopic lumbar discectomy results for 60 cases in professional and Olympic athletes.
Spine J. 2003 Mar-Apr;3(2):100-5.

An HS, Simpson JM, Stein R.: Outpatient laminotomy and discectomy.
J Spinal Disord. 1999 Jun;12(3):192-6.

Williams RW.: Microdiskectomy—myth, mania, or milestone? An 18-year surgical adventure.
Mt Sinai J Med. 1991 Mar;58(2):139-45.

Kambin P, Cohen LF.: Arthroscopic microdiscectomy versus nucleotomy techniques.
Clin Sports Med. 1993 Jul;12(3):587-98.

Donaldson WF 3rd, Star MJ, Thorne RP.: Surgical treatment for the far lateral herniated lumbar disc.
Spine. 1993 Aug;18(10):1263-7.

DeLuca PF, Mason DE, Weiand R, Howard R, Bassett GS.: Excision of herniated nucleus pulposus in children and adolescents.
J Pediatr Orthop. 1994 May-Jun;14(3):318-22.

Wong CH, Thng PL, Thoo FL, Low CO.: Symptomatic spinal epidural varices presenting with nerve impingement: report of two cases and review of the literature.
Spine. 2003 Sep 1;28(17):E347-50.

Girardi FP, Cammisa FP Jr, Huang RC, Parvataneni HK, Tsairis P.: Improvement of preoperative foot drop after lumbar surgery.
J Spinal Disord Tech. 2002 Dec;15(6):490-4.

Andreshak TG, An HS, Hall J, Stein B.Lumbar spine surgery in the obese patient.
J Spinal Disord. 1997 Oct;10(5):376-9.

Glasser RS, Knego RS, Delashaw JB, Fessler RG.: The perioperative use of corticosteroids and bupivacaine in the management of lumbar disc disease.
J Neurosurg. 1993 Mar;78(3):383-7.

McLain RF, Kalfas I, Bell GR, Tetzlaff JE, Yoon HJ, Rana M.: Comparison of spinal and general anesthesia in lumbar laminectomy surgery: a case-controlled analysis of 400 patients.
J Neurosurg Spine. 2005 Jan;2(1):17-22.

Mirzai H, Tekin I, Alincak H.: Perioperative use of corticosteroid and bupivacaine combination in lumbar disc surgery: a randomized controlled trial.
Spine. 2002 Feb 15;27(4):343-6.

DEGENERATIVE DISC DISEASE

Kader DF, Wardlaw D, Smith FW.: Correlation between the MRI changes in the lumbar multifidus muscles and leg pain.
Clin Radiol. 2000 Feb;55(2):145-9.

Cohen SP, Larkin TM, Barna SA, Palmer WE, Hecht AC, Stojanovic MP.: Lumbar discography: a comprehensive review of outcome studies, diagnostic accuracy, and principles.
Reg Anesth Pain Med. 2005 Mar-Apr;30(2):163-83.

Chen YC, Lee SH, Saenz Y, Lehman NL.: Histologic findings of disc, end plate and neural elements after coblation of nucleus pulposus: an experimental nucleoplasty study.
Spine J. 2003 Nov-Dec;3(6):466-70.

Huang RC, Lim MR, Girardi FP, Cammisa FP Jr.: The prevalence of contraindications to total disc replacement in a cohort of lumbar surgical patients.
Spine. 2004 Nov 15;29(22):2538-41.

RADIOFREQUENCY DENERVATION

Oh WS, Shim JC.: A randomized controlled trial of radiofrequency denervation of the ramus communicans nerve for chronic discogenic low back pain.
Clin J Pain. 2004 Jan-Feb;20(1):55-60.

IDET

Derby R, Seo KS, Kazala K, Chen YC, Lee SH, Kim BJ.: A factor analysis of lumbar intradiscal electrothermal annuloplasty outcomes.
Spine J. 2005 May-Jun;5(3):256-61.

Davis TT, Delamarter RB, Sra P, Goldstein TB.: The IDET procedure for chronic discogenic low back pain.
Spine. 2004 Apr 16;29(7):752-6.

Freedman BA, Cohen SP, Kuklo TR, Lehman RA, Larkin P, Giuliani JR.: Intradiscal electrothermal therapy (IDET) for chronic low back pain in active-duty soldiers: 2-year follow-up.
Spine J. 2003 Nov-Dec;3(6):502-9.

Spruit M, Jacobs WC.Pain and function after intradiscal electrothermal treatment (IDET) for symptomatic lumbar disc degeneration.
Eur Spine J. 2002 Dec;11(6):589-93. Epub 2002 Aug 9.

Saal JA, Saal JS.:Intradiscal electrothermal treatment for chronic discogenic low back pain: prospective outcome study with a minimum 2-year follow-up.
Spine. 2002 May 1;27(9):966-73; discussion 973-4.

PLIF

Ido K, Asada Y, Sakamoto T, Hayashi R, Kuriyama S.: Use of an autologous cortical bone graft sandwiched between two intervertebral spacers in posterior lumbar interbody fusion.
Neurosurg Rev. 2001 Jul;24(2-3):119-22.

Okuda S, Iwasaki M, Miyauchi A, Aono H, Morita M, Yamamoto T.:Risk factors for adjacent segment degeneration after PLIF.
Spine. 2004 Jul 15;29(14):1535-40. 1)

Brislin B, Vaccaro AR.: Advances in posterior lumbar interbody fusion.
Orthop Clin North Am. 2002 Apr;33(2):367-74.

TLIF

Schwender JD, Holly LT, Rouben DP, Foley KT.: Minimally invasive transforaminal lumbar interbody fusion (TLIF): technical feasibility and initial results.
J Spinal Disord Tech. 2005 Feb;18 Suppl:S1-6.

Hackenberg L, Halm H, Bullmann V, Vieth V, Schneider M, Liljenqvist U.:Transforaminal lumbar interbody fusion: a safe technique with satisfactory three to five year results.
Eur Spine J. 2005 Jan 26

Mummaneni PV, Pan J, Haid RW, Rodts GE.: Contribution of recombinant human bone morphogenetic protein-2 to the rapid creation of interbody fusion when used in transforaminal lumbar interbody fusion: a preliminary report. Invited submission from the Joint Section Meeting on Disorders of the Spine and Peripheral Nerves, March 2004.
J Neurosurg Spine. 2004 Jul;1(1):19-23.

O'Leary PF, McCance SE.: Distraction laminoplasty for decompression of lumbar spinal stenosis.
Clin Orthop Relat Res. 2001 Mar;(384)26-34

Sheehan JM, Shaffrey CI, Jane JA Sr.: Degenerative lumbar stenosis: the neurosurgical perspective.
Clin Orthop Relat Res. 2001 Mar;(384):61-74.

Yukawa Y, Lenke LG, Tenhula J, Bridwell KH, Riew KD, Blanke K.:
A comprehensive study of patients with surgically treated lumbar spinal stenosis with neurogenic claudication.
J Bone Joint Surg Am. 2002 Nov;84-A(11):1954-9.

Katz JN, Lipson SJ, Chang LC, Levine SA, Fossel AH, Liang MH.: Seven- to 10-year outcome of decompressive surgery for degenerative lumbar spinal stenosis.
Spine. 1996 Jan 1;21(1):92-8.

Chang Y, Singer DE, Wu YA, Keller RB, Atlas SJ.: The effect of surgical and nonsurgical treatment on longitudinal outcomes of lumbar spinal stenosis over 10 years.
J Am Geriatr Soc. 2005 May;53(5):785-92.

Atlas SJ, Keller RB, Wu YA, Deyo RA, Singer DE.: Long-term outcomes of surgical and nonsurgical management of lumbar spinal stenosis: 8 to 10 year results from the maine lumbar spine study.
Spine. 2005 Apr 15;30(8):936-43.

Jansson KA, Nemeth G, Granath F, Blomqvist P.: Spinal stenosis re-operation rate in Sweden is 11% at 10 years-A national analysis of 9,664 operations.
Eur Spine J. 2005 Mar 8

Wang MY, Green BA, Shah S, Vanni S, Levi AD.: Complications associated with lumbar stenosis surgery in patients older than 75 years of age.
Neurosurg Focus. 2003 Feb 15;14(2):e7.

Galiano K, Obwegeser AA, Gabl MV, Bauer R, Twerdy K.: Long-term outcome of laminectomy for spinal stenosis in octogenarians.
Spine. 2005 Feb 1;30(3):332-5.

Shabat S, Leitner Y, Nyska M, Berner Y, Fredman B, Gepstein R.Surgical treatment of lumbar spinal stenosis in patients aged 65 years and older.
Arch Gerontol Geriatr. 2002 Sep-Oct;35(2):143-52.

Hee HT, Wong HK.: The long-term results of surgical treatment for spinal stenosis in the elderly.
Singapore Med J. 2003 Apr;44(4):175-80.

Ragab AA, Fye MA, Bohlman HH: Surgery of the lumbar spine for spinal stenosis in 118 patients 70 years of age or older.
Spine. 2003 Feb 15;28(4):348-53.

Benz RJ, Ibrahim ZG, Afshar P, Garfin SR.: Predicting complications in elderly patients undergoing lumbar decompression.
Clin Orthop Relat Res. 2001 Mar;(384):116-21.

Does obesity affect the results of lumbar decompressive spinal surgery in the elderly? Gepstein R, Shabat S, Arinzon ZH, Berner Y, Catz A, Folman Y.
Clin Orthop Relat Res. 2004 Sep;(426):138-44.

Shapiro GS, Taira G, Boachie-Adjei O.: Results of surgical treatment of adult idiopathic scoliosis with low back pain and spinal stenosis: a study of long-term clinical radiographic outcomes.
Spine. 2003 Feb 15;28(4):358-63.

Simmons ED.: Surgical treatment of patients with lumbar spinal stenosis with associated scoliosis.
Clin Orthop Relat Res. 2001 Mar;(384):45-53.

Lee J, Hida K, Seki T, Iwasaki Y, Minoru A.An interspinous process distractor (X STOP) for lumbar spinal stenosis in elderly patients: preliminary experiences in 10 consecutive cases.
J Spinal Disord Tech. 2004 Feb;17(1):72-7; discussion 78.

MEDICAL EVALUATIONS FOR SPINAL SURGERY

Faciszewski T, Jensen R, Rokey R, Berg R.: Cardiac risk stratification of patients with symptomatic spinal stenosis.
Clin Orthop Relat Res. 2001 Mar;(384):110-5.

Reeg SE.: A review of comorbidities and spinal surgery.
Clin Orthop Relat Res. 2001 Mar;(384):101-9.

BLOODLESS STRATEGIES

Chillemi S, Sinardi D, Marino A, Mantarro G, Campisi R.The use of remifentanil for bloodless surgical field during vertebral disc resection.
Minerva Anestesiol. 2002 Sep;68(9):645-9.

Lee TC, Yang LC, Chen HJ.: Effect of patient position and hypotensive anesthesia on inferior vena caval pressure.
Spine. 1998 Apr 15;23(8):941-7; discussion 947-8.

Goodnough LT, Marcus RE.Effect of autologous blood donation in patients undergoing elective spine surgery.
Spine. 1992 Feb;17(2):172-5.

Keating EM.: Preoperative evaluation and methods to reduce blood use in orthopedic surgery.
Anesthesiol Clin North America. 2005 Jun;23(2):305-13.

Keating EM, Meding JB.: Perioperative blood management practices in elective orthopaedic surgery.
J Am Acad Orthop Surg. 2002 Nov-Dec;10(6):393-400.

Weber EW, Slappendel R, Hemon Y, Mahler S, Dalen T, Rouwet E, van Os J, Vosmaer A, van der Ark P.: Effects of epoetin alfa on blood transfusions and postoperative recovery in orthopaedic surgery: the European Epoetin Alfa Surgery Trial (EEST).
Eur J Anaesthesiol. 2005 Apr;22(4):249-57.

Koscielny J, Ziemer S, Radtke H, Schmutzler M, Pruss A, Sinha P, Salama A, Kiesewetter H, Latza R.: A practical concept for preoperative identification of patients with impaired primary hemostasis.
Clin Appl Thromb Hemost. 2004 Jul;10(3):195-204.

Houry S, Georgeac C, Hay JM, Fingerhut A, Boudet MJ.A prospective multicenter evaluation of preoperative hemostatic screening tests. The French Associations for Surgical Research.
Am J Surg. 1995 Jul;170(1):19-23.

Borzotta AP, Keeling MM.Value of the preoperative history as an indicator of hemostatic disorders.
Ann Surg. 1984 Nov;200(5):648-52.

Stovall TG.: Clinical experience with epoetin alfa in the management of hemoglobin levels in orthopedic surgery and cancer. Implications for use in gynecologic surgery.
J Reprod Med. 2001 May;46(5 Suppl):531-8.

Andrews CM, Lane DW, Bradley JG.: Iron pre-load for major joint replacement.
Transfus Med. 1997 Dec;7(4):281-6.

Bodnaruk ZM, Wong CJ, Thomas MJ.: Meeting the clinical challenge of care for Jehovah's Witnesses.
Transfus Med Rev. 2004 Apr;18(2):105-16.

Gohel MS, Bulbulia RA, Slim FJ, Poskitt KR, Whyman MR.: How to approach major surgery where patients refuse blood transfusion (including Jehovah's Witnesses).
Ann R Coll Surg Engl. 2005 Jan;87(1):3-14.

Winter RB, Swayze C.: Severe neurofibromatosis kyphoscoliosis in a Jehovah's Witness. Anterior and posterior spine fusion without blood transfusion.
Spine. 1983 Jan-Feb;8(1):39-42.

Guanciale AF, Dinsay JM, Watkins RG.: Lumbar lordosis in spinal fusion. A comparison of intraoperative results of patient positioning on two different operative table frame types.
Spine. 1996 Apr 15;21(8):964-9.

Weiss DS.: Spinal cord and nerve root monitoring during surgical treatment of lumbar stenosis.
Clin Orthop Relat Res. 2001 Mar;(384):82-100.

Voorhees JR, Cohen-Gadol AA, Laws ER, Spencer DD.: Battling blood loss in neurosurgery: Harvey Cushing's embrace of electrosurgery.
J Neurosurg. 2005 Apr;102(4):745-52.

Sugita K, Tsugane R.: Bipolar coagulator with automatic thermocontrol. Technical note.
J Neurosurg. 1974 Dec;41(6):777-9.

Cakir B, Ulmar B, Schmidt R, Kelsch G, Geiger P, Mehrkens HH, Puhl W, Richter M.: Efficacy and cost effectiveness of harmonic scalpel compared with electrocautery in posterior instrumentation of the spine.
Eur Spine J. 2005 Feb 15.

Majd ME, Farley S, Holt RT.: Preliminary outcomes and efficacy of the first 360 consecutive kyphoplasties for the treatment of painful osteoporotic vertebral compression fractures.
Spine J. 2005 May-Jun;5(3):244-55.

Takemasa R.:Vertebroplasty for osteoporotic vertebral compression fractures
Clin Calcium. 2003 Oct;13(10):1306-9.

Evans AJ, Jensen ME, Kip KE, DeNardo AJ, Lawler GJ, Negin GA, Remley KB, Boutin SM, Dunnagan SA.: Vertebral compression fractures: pain reduction and improvement in functional mobility after percutaneous polymethylmethacrylate vertebroplasty retrospective report of 245 cases.
Radiology. 2003 Feb;226(2):366-72.

Kaw LL Jr, Coimbra R, Potenza BM, Garfin SR, Hoyt DB.: The use of recombinant factor VIIa for severe intractable bleeding during spine surgery.
Spine. 2004 Jun 15;29(12):1384-7; discussion 1388.

Murray D.: Acute normovolemic hemodilution.
Eur Spine J. 2004 Oct;13 Suppl 1:S72-5. Epub 2004 Jun 10.

Sebastian C, Romero R, Olalla E, Ferrer C, Garcia-Vallejo JJ, Munoz M.: Postoperative blood salvage and reinfusion in spinal surgery: blood quality, effectiveness and impact on patient blood parameters.
Eur Spine J. 2000 Dec;9(6):458-65.

Cha CW, Deible C, Muzzonigro T, Lopez-Plaza I, Vogt M, Kang JD.: Allogeneic transfusion requirements after autologous donations in posterior lumbar surgeries.
Spine. 2002 Jan 1;27(1):99-104.

Kobayashi K.: Artificial blood
Nippon Geka Gakkai Zasshi. 2005 Jan;106(1):31-7.